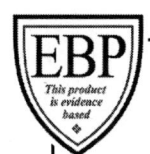

Evidence-Based Competency Management *for the* Medical-Surgical Unit

SECOND EDITION

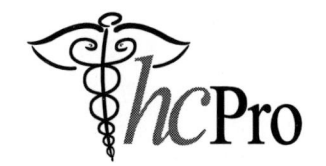

hcPro

Evidence-Based Competency Management for the Medical-Surgical Unit, Second Edition, is published by HCPro, Inc.

Copyright © 2008, 2005 HCPro, Inc.

All rights reserved. Printed in the United States of America.   5 4 3 2 1

First edition published 2005. Second edition published 2008.

ISBN: 978-1-60146-154-4

No part of this publication may be reproduced, in any form or by any means, without prior written consent of HCPro, Inc., or the Copyright Clearance Center (978/750-8400). Please notify us immediately if you have received an unauthorized copy.

HCPro, Inc., provides information resources for the healthcare industry.

HCPro, Inc., is not affiliated in any way with The Joint Commission, which owns the JCAHO and Joint Commission trademarks. MAGNET™, MAGNET RECOGNITION PROGRAM®, and ANCC MAGNET RECOGNITION® are trademarks of the American Nurses Credentialing Center (ANCC). The products and services of HCPro, Inc., and The Greeley Company are neither sponsored nor endorsed by the ANCC.

Barbara A. Brunt, MA, MN, RN-BC, Author
Adrianne E. Avillion, DEd, RN, Contributing Author
Gwen A. Valois, MS, RN, BC, Contributing Author
Jane G. Alberico, MS, RN, CEN, Contributing Author
Emily Sheahan, Group Publisher
Rebecca Hendren, Senior Managing Editor
Lindsey Cardarelli, Associate Editor
Audrey Doyle, Copyeditor

Janell Lukac, Layout Artist
Crystal Beland, Layout Artist
Patrick Campagnone, Cover Designer
Liza Banks, Proofreader
Darren Kelly, Books Production Supervisor
Susan Darbyshire, Art Director
Claire Cloutier, Production Manager
Jean St. Pierre, Director of Operations

Advice given is general. Readers should consult professional counsel for specific legal, ethical, or clinical questions.

Arrangements can be made for quantity discounts. For more information, contact:

HCPro, Inc.
P.O. Box 1168
Marblehead, MA 01945
Telephone: 800/650-6787 or 781/639-1872
Fax: 781/639-2982
E-mail: *customerservice@hcpro.com*

Visit HCPro at its World Wide Web sites: *www.hcpro.com* **and** *www.hcmarketplace.com*

Contents

List of figures v

About the author vi

About the contributing authors vii

Preface ix
    Step 1: Gather applicant information x
    Step 2: Verify the applicant's information xi
    Step 3: Continually verify the employee's license after the hire date xii

How to use this book xiii

How to use the files on your CD-ROM xvi

Introduction xxii

Chapter 1: Why is competency validation required? 1
    Regulating competence 3
    The Joint Commission 7
    Competency and litigation 15

Chapter 2: What is competency validation? 19
    Competency-based education 21
    Defining competencies 30
    Classifying competencies by domains and levels 30
    Who performs competency validation? 32
    Mandatory training versus competencies 32
    Mapping competencies for orientation, annual assessments 34
    Methods for validating competencies 36

Chapter 3: Competency validation in job descriptions and performance evaluations 41
    The benefits 44
    The Joint Commission's expectations 45
    Key elements of a competency-based job description 46

Contents

Chapter 4: Train the staff to perform competency validation 53
- Developing a competency assessment training program 56
- Identifying your competency assessors 59
- Peer review 63
- Keeping your validation system consistent 64
- Incorporating population-specific competencies 66
- Documentation and recordkeeping 72
- Conclusion 73

Chapter 5: Keep up with new competencies 75
- Potential categories for new competencies 78
- Interpersonal communications 78
- Guidelines for new competency development 80
- Best practices for the implementation of new competencies 85
- Dimensions of competencies 88

Chapter 6: Using your skills checklists 91
- Differences between orientation checklists and skills checklists 97
- Skills checklists for annual competency assessment 112

ALL: General, All Units 119

MS: Medical-Surgical 151

ROLE: Role Related 315

Bibliography 365

Nursing education instructional guide 371

List of figures

Figure 2.1: Comparison of CBE and traditional education 22
Figure 2.2: Sample competency-based program policy 24
Figure 3.1: Essential functions..48
Figure 3.2: Rating scale and definitions..50
Figure 4.1: Successful completion of competency assessment training form 62
Figure 4.2: Case Studies 68
Figure 5.1: New competency assessment checklist..83
Figure 6.1: Skills checklist template...95
Figure 6.2: Competency-based orientation checklist..98
Figure 6.3: Nursing assistant orientation checklist...105
Figure 6.4: Competencies tracking sheet 114

About the author

Barbara A. Brunt, MA, MN, RN-BC

Barbara A. Brunt, MA, MN, RN-BC, is Director of Nursing Education and Staff Development for Summa Health System in Akron, OH. She has held a variety of staff development position, including educator, coordinator, and director for the past 30 years. Brunt has presented on a variety of topics both locally and nationally, and has published numerous articles, chapters in books, and books. She served as a section editor for all three editions of the *Core Curriculum for Staff Development* published by the National Nursing Staff Development Organization (NNSDO) and coauthored a book *Nursing Professional Development: Nursing Review and Resource Manual*, published by the American Nurses Credentialing Center Institute for Credentialing Innovation. She was the author of *Competencies for Staff Educators: Tools to Evaluate and Enhance Nursing Professional Development*, published by HCPro, Inc.

Brunt holds a master's degree in community health education from Kent State University and a master's degree in nursing from the University of Dundee in Scotland. Her research has focused on competencies. Brunt maintains certification in Nursing Professional Development and has been active in numerous professional associations. She is currently serving a two-year term as President of NNSDO, and a term as second vice-president for the Delta Omega Chapter of Sigma Theta Tau International. She has received awards for excellence in writing, nursing research, leadership, and staff development.

About the contributing authors

Adrianne E. Avillion, DEd, RN

Adrianne E. Avillion, DEd, RN, is the owner of Avillion's Curriculum Design in York, PA. She specializes in designing continuing education programs for healthcare professionals and freelance medical writing. She also offers consulting services in work redesign, quality improvement, and staff development.

Avillion has published extensively, including serving as editor of the first and second editions of *The Core Curriculum for Staff Development*. Her most recent publications include *Evidence-Based Staff Development: Strategies to Create, Measure, and Refine Your Program, A Practical Guide to Staff Development: Tools and Techniques for Effective Education,* and *Designing Nursing Orientation: Evidence-Based Strategies for Effective Programs*, all published by HCPro, Inc. in Marblehead, MA, and *Nurse Entrepreneurship: The Art of Running Your Own Business*, published by Creative Health Care Management in Minneapolis, MN. She is also a frequent presenter at conferences and conventions devoted to the specialty of continuing education and staff development.

Gwen A. Valois, MS, RN, BC

Gwen A. Valois, MS, RN, BC, is the director of organizational development at Medical City Dallas Hospital in Dallas. She has clinical expertise in pediatrics and has served for more than 25 years in various clinical educational and leadership roles.

Valois received her BSN from Texas Woman's University, her master's degree in human resource management and development from National Louis University, and holds certification from the American Nurses Credentialing Center in nursing professional development.

About the contributing authors

Jane G. Alberico, MS, RN, CEN

Jane G. Alberico, MS, RN, CEN, has more than 30 years of nursing practice in healthcare. She received her bachelor's of science degree from the University of Kentucky and master's degree in health science instruction, with a minor in healthcare administration, from Texas Woman's University.

Alberico is a certified emergency nurse whose clinical expertise includes medical-surgical, home health, pain management, and emergency care. She has served in faculty and leadership roles in school and hospital settings. She is a national speaker for various topics and is currently the supervisor for clinical education at Medical City Dallas Hospital in Dallas.

Preface

Before you use any methodology for validating and assessing the competency of your nurses to deliver safe patient care, it is essential that you have a system in place for verifying that your nurses are who they say they are prior to allowing them on your units.

This might sound obvious, but stories of nurses faking credentials, hopping from job to job in various states, and harming patients are stark reminders that you must be diligent in verifying any nursing applicant's licensure, criminal background, education, and employment history.

Nurse-credentialing processes at some facilities may be inadequate. Nurses who have had action taken against them by another state nursing board, have a criminal history, or have incomplete education may slip by and end up working in direct contact with your patients, making those patients vulnerable and your facility liable. You should examine your organization's policies to make sure they protect your patients, and sufficiently screen applicants for dangerous nurses or imposters.

Credentialing nurses falls to the HR department in most facilities, and the medical staff office handles physician and advance-practice RN credentialing. For advice on credentialing nurses, HR administrators can consult their colleagues in the medical staff office, who most likely already have an established credentialing process in place.

Here are some steps you can take to verify nurses' credentials and to ensure your patients' safety and your facility's integrity.

Step 1: Gather applicant information

The application for employment should be thorough and should obtain the information needed to ensure patient safety in your facility. Ask for the following:

- The applicant's name and any other names he or she has used (e.g., a maiden name)
- Education, the degree obtained, and the name and location of the educational institution
- Professional licensure, the state in which the license was issued, the date issued, the license number, and the expiration date
- Disciplinary actions on the license
- Specialty certification
- Employment history

With many new nursing schools starting up, the organization needs to determine whether it requires nursing applicants to be graduates of an accredited school of nursing. New programs cannot apply for National League for Nursing Accreditation Commission accreditation until after their first class has graduated, which means that organizations that require graduation from an accredited school cannot hire any graduates of these programs.

That also requires that the accreditation status of all schools from which a potential applicant graduated must be verified prior to hire. Is licensure to practice as a nurse in that state sufficient? Whatever policy the organization decides to follow must be followed consistently, and must be reflected in the job descriptions.

It is also important to determine whether the applicant has even been convicted or pleaded guilty or no contest to the following:

- Criminal charges (other than speeding violations)
- Drug- or alcohol-related offenses

If either one of these situations applies, ask the applicant to specify the charges and the dates on which they occurred. Finally, inquire whether he or she has ever been suspended, sanctioned, or otherwise restricted from participating in any private, federal, or state health insurance program (e.g., Medicare or Medicaid) or similar federal, state, or health agency.

Step 2: Verify the applicant's information

Verify to the best of your ability the information you obtained on the application. Even if you don't find anything, document each verification step to further reduce your hospital's liability.

Some facilities hire a third party to verify this information, but most often the HR department performs this task. Either way, make sure a specific, established process is in place.

The best method of checking an applicant's qualifications is to use primary source verification, including education, licensure, and past employment. For the most accurate and up-to-date information, you should check the state board in every state that the applicant nurse has worked. Most state licensing boards post licensure information on their Web sites.

Many organizations require criminal background checks on all applicants, even if the state nursing board runs checks on its own. Nurses may have committed a crime after receiving their licenses. In most states, the responsibility is on nurses to notify the state board it they are convicted of a crime, but they may or may not do so, which puts your facility at risk.

Another important part of the process is to check federal sanctions lists. If you hire a nurse who has been sanctioned by the Office of Inspector General or General Services Administration, you could be fined thousands of dollars. Reasons for sanctions include everything from defaulting on student loans to Medicare fraud.

Here are some other potential "red flags" to consider:

- **Gaps in job history:** HR professionals are well aware of this red flag, but be sure to ask about the gaps. Understand that there could be a perfectly good explanation, such as the birth of a child or a family emergency.

- **Moving from state to state:** When an applicant moves around a lot, his or her licensure information could be buried or lost. Therefore, be sure to check the status of the license in each state in which the applicant practiced.

- **Job hopping:** HR professionals are well aware of this pattern as well, and they will look twice at any applicant with evidence of it. But be sure to call each employer and verify that no disciplinary actions were taken against the applicant.

Step 3: Continually verify the employee's license after the hire date

Most facilities check nurses' licenses when they are up for renewal to make sure they are current and active. However, it is crucial that you institute a process to verify licensure status more often as well.

Ensure that your policy spells out that it is the nurse's responsibility to report any disciplinary action taken against his or her license over the course of his or her employment. If your nurses do not report such action, they could be working on your unit with a suspended or inactive license and you would have no idea. Many boards of nursing post disciplinary actions against nurses in that state, which can be used as another method to ensure that all employees have a current license with no restriction.

Creating a new credential-verification process or updating your current process is a very important prerequisite to the competency assessment process.

How to use this book

Evidence-Based Competency Management for the Medical-Surgical Unit, Second Edition, will help you understand the basics of competency validation and assessment and discuss the steps you need to take to develop a process for performing these assessments at your organization.

In addition, this book provides you with evidence-based sample tools that will help get you started.

The appendix contains 122 evidence-based sample competency validation skill sheets. The skill sheets are organized into two sections: General and Medical-Surgical. In addition, the appendix contains 24 role-related checklists, which can be used for orientation, training, or review purposes. The first page of each section contains a table of contents, which lists the name and page number of each skill sheet included in that section.

All of the content in the skill sheets was contributed or updated by Summa Health System Hospitals in Akron, OH. This content has been reprinted with the permission of this organization.

Customizable, electronic versions of all the skill sheets can be found on the CD-ROM accompanying the book. We have also included a copy of the "Competencies Analyzer" on your CD-ROM. This easy-to-use spreadsheet will help your unit or department managers organize their competency assessment program. A complete list of tools included on the CD-ROM can be found in the "How to use the CD-ROM section."

Putting your skill sheets to work

The template used to standardize the appearance of these skills sheets appears on your CD-ROM. Save this blank template to your computer and use it to create additional skill sheets for your organization.

Duplicate this blank sheet as many times as needed. Type in content as you would into any table created using Microsoft's word-processing software to customize the sheets to fit your organization's needs, using the information discussed in this manual.

How to use this book

Here is a quick look at one of the skill sheets:

Name, date, skill – the section includes a space for the name of the employee whose competency is being validated, the date the validation is taking place, and the name of the skill being validated. Consider adding a second identifier, such as the employee number, to this section.

We have already provided the name of the skills for each of the skill sheets included in the manual. As we discuss in Chapter 2, however, all the competencies validated by your organization will not be technical or skill-based competencies, such as using a blood-glucose meter. Therefore, when customizing these sheets for validation on an interpersonal competency or a cultural competency, consider changing the term "skill" to "behavior" as a more accurate way to incorporate the elected required of these competencies.

Steps, completed, comments – This section is set up in a typical checklist format. After each step is successfully completed, the validator would add a check to the "completed" column. Consider changing the term "steps" to "performance criteria" when creating sheets for competencies that may not conform to a step-by-step format. The validator can use the "comments" column to record statements such as "needs reinforcement for steps" or "reteaching required."

Self-assessment – The validator should ask the employee to do a self-assessment of his or her competence on the skill being validated. Use this section to check off the appropriate response.

Evaluation/validation methods – This box contains some of the more common methodologies used to validate competencies. The validator should note which method was used in association with the skill sheet to validate the competency.

Levels – Consideration for the level of proficiency should be made when validating competencies (refer to Chapter 2). The level of proficiency (i.e., beginner, intermediate, expert) should coincide with the experience level of the employee. Should the level not coincide, then remediation should be planned to achieve the desired level of competence.

Type of validation – In this section, the validator can specify whether this competency validation tool was used during orientation, during an annual competency assessment, or at another point during the competency validation process.

Employee observer signature – Have both the employee and the validator (i.e., observer) sign the completed tool. This helps ensure the employee was an active participant in the process and that he or she understands and acknowledges this piece of the competency validation process.

How to use the files on your CD-ROM

The following file names correspond with figures listed in the book, *Evidence-Based Competency Management for the Medical-Surgical Unit, Second Edition.*

sstemp.rtf	Blank skillsheet template
analyze.xls	Competencies Analyzer
Fig3-1.rtf	Figure 3.1: Essential functions
Fig4-1.rtf	Figure 4.1: Successful completion of competency assessment training form
Fig5-1.rtf	Figure 5.1: New competency assessment checklist
Fig6-2.rtf	Figure 6.2: Competency-based orientation checklist
Fig6-3.rtf	Figure 6.3: Nursing assistant orientation checklist

General:

General1.rtf	ABG Interpretation
General2.rtf	Annual Competency Performance—Quality of Instruction
General3.rtf	Arjo Ceiling Lift
General4.rtf	Assessment/Validation of Competencies
General5.rtf	Assisting Adult with Feeding
General6.rtf	Blood Glucose Meter
General7.rtf	Blood Pressure Measurement – Automatic
General8.rtf	Blood Pressure Measurement – Manual
General9.rtf	Digital Holter Hookup (Diagnostic Cardiology)
General10.rtf	Emergency Preparedness
General11.rtf	Falls Prevention (Get Up and Go)
General12.rtf	Fit Testing for N-95 Respirator Mask
General13.rtf	Intake and Output
General14.rtf	Medication Administration
General15.rtf	Oxygen Administration
General16.rtf	Presentation Skills

General17.rtf	Regulating and Monitoring IV Rate
General18.rtf	Service Excellence
General19.rtf	Thrombolytic Therapy
General20.rtf	Thrombus, Chronic versus Acute
General21.rtf	Use of Automated External Defibrillator (Heartstream FR2)
General22.rtf	Venipuncture with Winged Needle

Medical-Surgical Unit:

Ms1.rtf	Accessing Implantable Access Devices
Ms2.rtf	Adding IV Solution, Priming Tubing, Changing Tubing
Ms3.rtf	Adding IV Solution to Central Line
Ms4.rtf	Administration of Blood
Ms5.rtf	Applanation Tonometry
Ms6.rtf	Appointment Scheduling – Clinic
Ms7.rtf	Atrium Ocean
Ms8.rtf	Barthel Index
Ms9.rtf	Bed Bath
Ms10.rtf	BICAP and Cautery
Ms11.rtf	Bladder Scanner
Ms12.rtf	Blood Culture Collection
Ms13.rtf	Braden Scale
Ms14.rtf	CADD Pump
Ms15.rtf	Care of Patient with Central Venous Catheter
Ms16.rtf	Central Venous Catheter – Application of Sterile Occlusive Dressing
Ms17.rtf	Central Venous Catheter – Obtaining Blood Samples
Ms18.rtf	Central Venous Catheter Removal
Ms19.rtf	Chemotherapy Administration
Ms20.rtf	Chemotherapy Teaching
Ms21.rtf	Chest Drainage Autotransfusion – Atrium Unit
Ms22.rtf	Chest Tube Dressing Change
Ms23.rtf	Code Management – Med/Surg
Ms24.rtf	Conscious Sedation

How to use the files on your CD-ROM

Ms25.rtf	Conversion to Intermittent Infusion of Continuous IV
Ms26.rtf	Crutch Walking and Use of Walker
Ms27.rtf	Discontinuing Intravenous (IV) Therapy
Ms28.rtf	Drug Testing (Blood and Urine)
Ms29.rtf	Flex Pen Patient Self-Administration
Ms30.rtf	GemStar Pump
Ms31.rtf	Homegoing Instructions
Ms32.rtf	Hypodermoclysis
Ms33.rtf	Infusion Intravenous Piggyback Administration (IVPB)
Ms34.rtf	Inline Tracheobronchial Sunction
Ms35.rtf	Insertion of Dobbhoff Feeding Tube
Ms36.rtf	Insulin Administration
Ms37.rtf	Insulin Administration Instruction
Ms38.rtf	Intramuscular Injections
Ms39.rtf	Intravenous Catheters – Declotting
Ms40.rtf	IV Dressing Changes
Ms41.rtf	IV Site – Drawing Blood From
Ms42.rtf	IV Start – Hemodialysis Catheter
Ms43.rtf	IV Starts and PRN adapter
Ms44.rtf	IV Therapy Documentation
Ms45.rtf	Lab Specimen Labeling Compliance
Ms46.rtf	Lidocaine for Insertion of IV Catheter
Ms47.rtf	Maintenance of Hickman Catheter
Ms48.rtf	Metered Dose Inhaler (MDI)
Ms49.rtf	Nasogastric Tube Maintenance
Ms50.rtf	Nasopharyngeal Suctioning
Ms51.rtf	Neurological Assessment and Documentation
Ms52.rtf	Neurovascular Status
Ms53.rtf	Neutropenic Precautions
Ms54.rtf	NIH Stroke Scale, Completing the National Institute of Health
Ms55.rtf	Normal Saline Wet to Dry Dressing
Ms56.rtf	Ocular Medication Administration

Ms57.rtf	Ophthalmic Medication Administration
Ms58.rtf	Oral Care of the Cancer Patient
Ms59.rtf	Patient Controlled Analgesia (PCA) Infuser
Ms60.rtf	Peripheral Blood Draw
Ms61.rtf	PICC Line – Applying a PRN Adapter
Ms62.rtf	PICC Line – Obtaining Blood samples
Ms63.rtf	PICC Line – Removing the PICC
Ms64.rtf	PICC Lines – Starting and Discontinuing an Infusion
Ms65.rtf	PICC Line- Suturing
Ms66.rtf	Pin Care
Ms67.rtf	Postoperative Assessment
Ms68.rtf	Presentation of Patient at Team Rounds
Ms69.rtf	Pulse Oximeter Monitor
Ms70.rtf	Pyxis Access
Ms71.rtf	Radial Artery Assessment
Ms72.rtf	Rehab Unit Transfer Techniques
Ms73.rtf	Restraints – Role of Nursing Assistants
Ms74.rtf	Seclusion Restraint (Behavioral Health)
Ms75.rtf	Skin Burn – Care of
Ms76.rtf	Skin Prep Using Tincture of Iodine
Ms77.rtf	Staple.Clip Removal
Ms78.rtf	Sterile Gloves, Applying
Ms79.rtf	Sterile Technique
Ms80.rtf	Subcutaneous Needle Placement
Ms81.rtf	Tenckhoff Catheter
Ms82.rtf	Tissue Therapy
Ms83.rtf	Tracheal Suctioning
Ms84.rtf	Tracheostomy Care
Ms85.rtf	Tracheostomy Tube Dislodgement, Emergency Intervention
Ms86.rtf	Transfer of Patient with Cervical Surgery and Patient with Shoulder Surgery
Ms87.rtf	Transfer Patient with Lumbar Surgery
Ms88.rtf	Transfer, Transport, Ambulation

How to use the files on your CD-ROM

Ms89.rtf	Transportation of Postcatheterization Patients
Ms90.rtf	Tuberculosis Skin Test
Ms91.rtf	Urinary Catheterization
Ms92.rtf	VAC: Negative Pressure Wound Therapy
Ms93.rtf	VACD (Vacuum Assisted Closure Device for Negative Pressure Wound Therapy)
Ms94.rtf	Venous Reflux Exam
Ms95.rtf	Ventilator, Assessment and Troubleshooting
Ms96.rtf	Vital Signs (Observation Room)
Ms97.rtf	Weights/Height – Digital
Ms98.rtf	Wound Culture
Ms99.rtf	Wound Photography
Ms100.rtf	Zoladex, Subcutaneous Injection of

Role Related:

Role1.rtf	Acid Mixing
Role2.rtf	Adding Toner to Fax
Role3.rtf	Administrative Associate Accurate Charging
Role4.rtf	Appointment Scheduling – Diabetes Center
Role5.rtf	Age-Specific Competency Checklist RN/LPN
Role6.rtf	Age-Specific Competency Checklist SA/AA
Role7.rtf	Behavioral Health Associate Skills Assessment/Evaluation
Role8.rtf	Bicarb Mixing
Role9.rtf	Charge Entry
Role10.rtf	Charge Nurse Assessment/Evaluation
Role11.rtf	Defibrillator Function — Daily Check (Lifepak 9)
Role12.rtf	Discharge Bed/Bassinette Cleaning for Environmental Associates
Role13.rtf	Hospital Outpatient Profile (HOP) Charges
Role14.rtf	Insurance Precertification Authorization
Role15.rtf	LPN Skills Assessment/Evaluation
Role16.rtf	Nursing Assistant Orientation Skills Assessment/Evaluation
Role17.rtf	Nursing Student Technician Competency Checklist
Role18.rtf	Private Duty RN/LPN Competency Evaluation

Role19.rtf	Registration
Role20.rtf	RN Skills Assessment/Evaluation
Role21.rtf	Sitter Guidelines
Role22.rtf	Telephone Skills
Role23.rtf	Telephone Skills (Problem Solving)
Role24.rtf	Unit Secretary Skills Assessment/Evaluation

To adapt any of the files to your own facility, simply follow the instructions below to open the CD.

If you have trouble reading the forms, click on "View," and then "Normal." To adapt the forms, save them first to your own hard drive or disk (by clicking "File," then "Save as," and changing the system to your own). Then change the information to fit your facility, and add or delete any items that you wish to change.

Installation instructions

This product was designed for the Windows operating system and includes Word files that will run under Windows 95/98 or greater. The CD will work on all PCs and most Macintosh systems. To run the files on the CD/ROM, take the following steps:

1. Insert the CD into your CD/ROM drive.
2. Double-click on the "My Computer" icon, next double-click on the CD drive icon.
3. Double-click on the files you wish to open.
4. Adapt the files by moving the cursor over the areas you wish to change, highlighting them, and typing in the new information using Microsoft Word.
5. To save a file to your facility's system, click on "File" and then click on "Save As." Select the location where you wish to save the file and then click on "Save."
6. To print a document, click on "File" and then click on "Print."

Introduction

The focus on competence and evidence-based practice (EBP) is pervasive in healthcare today. Not only do the various regulatory agencies require assessment and documentation of competence of staff members, but the expectation is that organizations use evidence-based practice to provide quality care.

EBP is the process of making clinical decisions based on the most current and valid research and high-quality data available, with the goal of improving patient safety and decreasing the number of medical errors (Avillion 2007).

The second edition of this book includes the evidence for all the competencies that are provided. It should not be assumed that the competencies in the first edition were not based on current literature or evidence, but that information was not included on the competency itself. In this edition, the evidence base for each competency is included as part of the competency itself.

For the second edition, information in all the chapters has been updated to provide current resources on the competency management process. Chapter 1 outlines why competency validation is required, Chapter 2 defines competency validation, and Chapter 3 discusses including information on why competency validation should be a part of job descriptions and the performance-evaluation process. Chapter 4 focuses on the training needed for staff to perform competency validation, and Chapter 5 provides suggestions on keeping up with new competencies. How to use the skills checklists is described in Chapter 6.

There are 146 competency validation skills sheets included in this edition. Some of the skills in the first edition were deleted and others were added based on current practice and best evidence. In addition to the categories included in the first edition, there is another category added for general checklists that are role-related. These bonus checklists focus on specific skills required of various care providers, so these do not include references. The checklists can be adapted for the specific needs of your organization.

I hope you find the information in this second edition helpful whether you are developing a competency management program or refining ones you currently have in place.

REFERENCES

1. Avillion, Adrianne E. (2007). *Evidence-Based Staff Development: Strategies to Create, Measure, and Refine Your Program.* Marblehead, MA: HCPro, Inc.

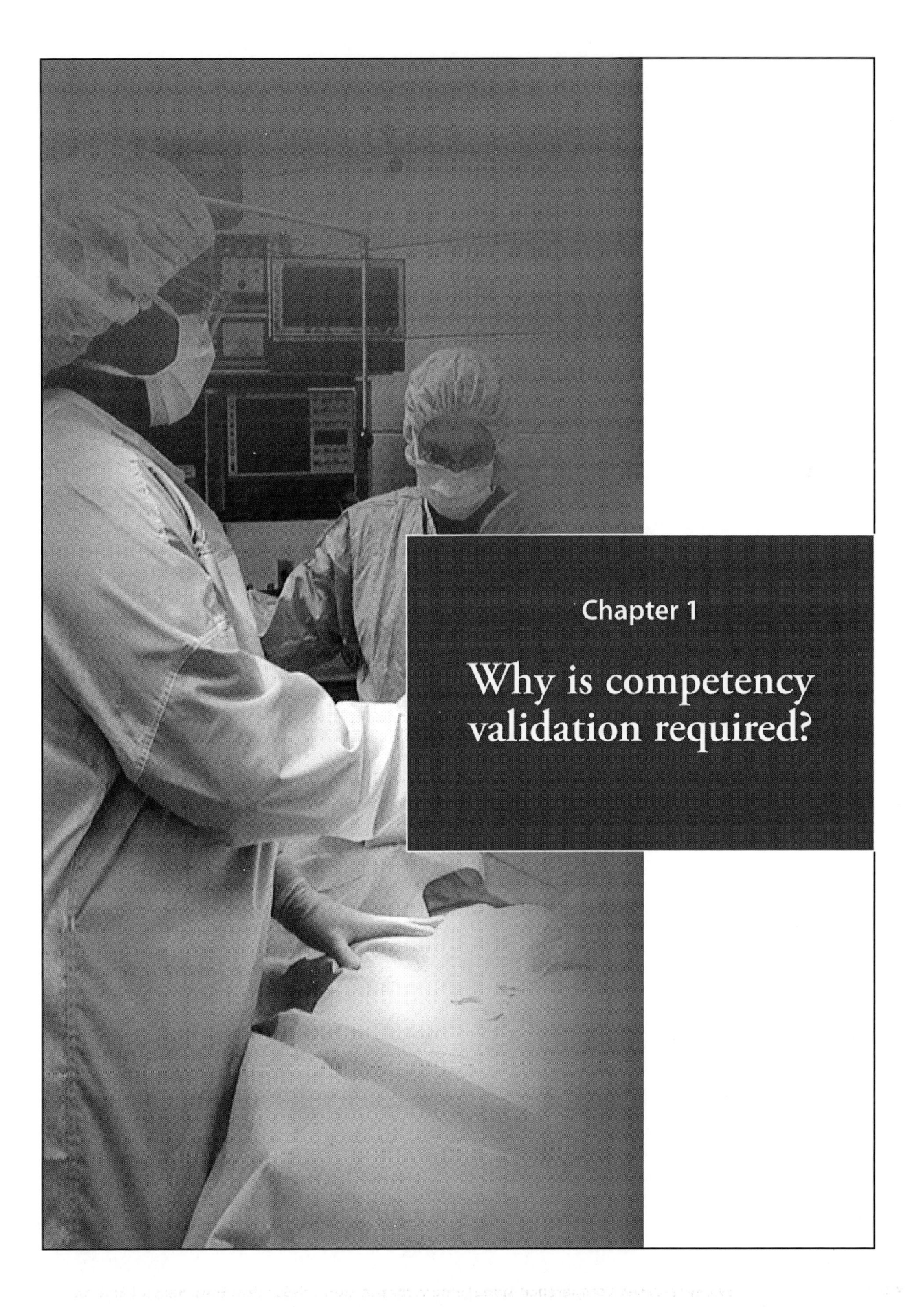

Chapter 1

Why is competency validation required?

Chapter 1

Why is competency validation required?

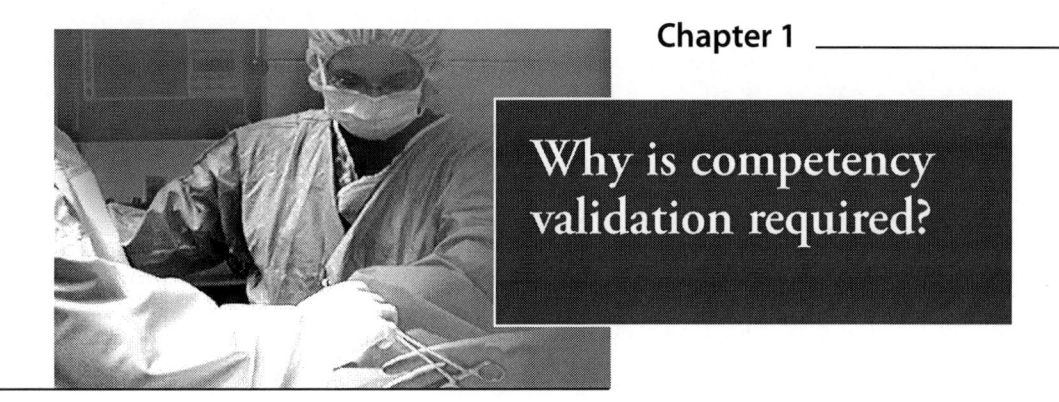

Learning objectives

After reading this chapter, the participant should be able to:

- Design a competency plan to effectively assess employee competence

Regulating competence

Does it seem as though regulatory survey teams visit you every day? Sometimes the survey is announced and sometimes it's a surprise, but every time, the surveyors—regardless of whom they represent—are concerned about "competency."

The definition of this word is in the eye of the beholder. *Webster's New World College Dictionary*, for instance, defines *competent* as "well qualified, capable, fit" (Agnes 2006). The American Nurses Association (ANA) defines *competency* as "an expected level of performance that results from an integration of knowledge, skills, abilities, and judgment" (ANA 2007). In healthcare, however, it's not so simple. Your healthcare staff make decisions and carry out responsibilities and job duties that affect patients' lives. When the goal is to achieve positive patient outcomes—whether to cure or manage a chronic disease process, or to allow someone to die a dignified death—will "sufficient ability" be good enough? Should competency apply only to clinical bedside nursing? Should an RN case manager have to meet the same competency requirements as a critical-care staff nurse? No, no, and no.

Chapter 1

Evidence-based practice involves supporting your actions with research and data, and basing competencies in evidence is becoming the standard in competency validation. Researchers have identified best practices for patient care based on evidence, so when assessing staff members' competence, they should be assessed based on their provision of evidence-based care. By instituting evidence-based practice in your competency assessment, you ensure the methods by which you are validating your staff members' skills are established and grounded in research. In this book, you are provided with references to the original research so you are able to institute evidence-based competency assessment at your facility.

Protecting the public

Regulatory agencies are rampant in the healthcare industry. Their purpose is to protect the public and to ensure a consistent standard of care for patients and families. Initially, there was only the Joint Commission on Accreditation of Hospitals (JCAH). Ernest Codman, a physician, proposed the standardization process for hospitals in 1910, and the American College of Surgeons developed the Minimum Standards for Hospitals in 1917 and officially transferred its program to the JCAH in 1952. A trickling of new agencies followed, and in 1964, the JCAH started charging for surveys. JCAH changed its name to the Joint Commission on Accreditation of Healthcare Organizations (JCAHO) in 1987 and is now known simply as The Joint Commission (The Joint Commission 2007).

The list of regulators today now looks like an alphabet soup. Political debates regarding the effectiveness of these agencies have multiplied in recent years. In July 2004, for example, the Centers for Medicare & Medicaid Services (CMS) began to criticize the validity of Joint Commission accreditations. However, since its inception, The Joint Commission has never had federal oversight (Knight 2004). In some cases, criteria for federally mandated CMS regulatory standards may exceed those of The Joint Commission.

For acute-care facilities, the agencies that "oversee" patient care and thus require competency assessment may now include the following:

- The Joint Commission
- CMS
- National Quality Foundation
- The Leapfrog Group

- State departments of health and human services
- State medical foundations
- ANA
- State Board of Nurse Examiners (BNE)
- Health Quality Improvement Initiatives
- Occupational Safety & Health Administration (OSHA)
- College of American Pathologists (CAP)
- Office of Inspector General
- Quality improvement organizations
- Agency for Healthcare Research and Quality
- The U.S. Food and Drug Administration
- Centers for Disease Control and Prevention (CDC)

Add to this a list of your hospital's competency assessment initiatives. Most of these initiatives revolve around the mission, vision, and value statements for the organization. Indicators may include:

- Patient satisfaction
- Physician satisfaction
- Employee health and pride
- Fiscal responsibility
- Community involvement
- Risk management

Those of us working in healthcare started our careers wanting to improve human life, and it is frustrating at times when it seems that the bureaucracy of regulatory mandates keeps growing. But the business of healthcare must consist of personnel who are both caring and able to perform their jobs safely and correctly. Remember that the provision of quality care and services depends on knowledgeable, competent healthcare providers. Every organization should have a competency plan in place to ensure that performance expectations based on job-specific position descriptions are consistently met.

You must design your competency plan with consideration given to:

- The mission, vision, and values of your organization
- The needs of patients and families served
- The extended community
- New services or technologies planned for future services
- Special needs required for particular healthcare situations
- Current standards of professional practice
- Applicable legal and regulatory agency requirements
- Organizational policies and procedures

In addition, the organization should foster learning on a continual basis. The CEO and nurse executive should mandate this learning environment and hold the leadership team and staff accountable for expected outcomes (Joint Commission Resources 2008). The entire organization must foster a work environment that helps employees discover what they need to learn for self-growth.

What's the return on this investment? A positive patient/family outcome. The outcome may be improved health, the ability to manage a chronic disorder, or even a dignified death.

A consistent process for competency assessment is essential throughout the organization for all job classes, contract personnel, and, when indicated, affiliating schools. There must be a centralized, organized approach that moves seamlessly throughout the continuum of care and ensures the same standard or practice for all of the patients and families it serves. If your main policies and procedures say one thing but certain departments or units develop their own policies and procedures that say something else, you are in trouble.

Generating tons of paperwork does not ensure competency in practice. Use the KISS method: "Keep it simple, smarty." Although documenting that standards are being met is important, regulatory surveyors are moving away from looking at paper. The trend is to interview patients, staff members, physicians, vendors, and members of the leadership team to see evidence of compliance. And now more than ever, there are expectations to move beyond merely verifying whether nurses are "competent." Thanks in part to advances in technology, nurses have been catapulted into more advanced and specialized care. Entire nursing divisions in hospital settings may now apply for American Nurses Credentialing Center (ANCC) Magnet Recognition Program® designation. Designations such as this and the Malcolm Baldrige National Quality Award are raising the bar for practice by empowering nurses to demand excellence in delivering care.

Instead of telling you months in advance the date on which it will arrive at your hospital, the regulatory agency may show up at your door at any time without advance notice. In fact, Joint Commission surveyors began doing so in 2006. Therefore, it is vital for you and your organization to be survey-ready every day. Ongoing performance must be measured and assessed. If individual members of your healthcare organization do not meet the standards you've established, individuals and the leadership team must develop a system for ongoing validation and assessment of personnel based on those standards. Remember: Competency assessment would be necessary even if it were not an accreditation standard.

It is worth framing this discussion on the expectations of regulatory agencies, because understanding their motivations and complying with their recommendations will result in a better understanding of what an effective competency assessment process should look like. What do these regulatory agencies want? In our upcoming discussion of The Joint Commission, we will also introduce the concepts of other state and federal agencies.

The Joint Commission

The Joint Commission is still considered to be the leader in healthcare accreditation. Standards devoted to competency are woven through The Joint Commission's accreditation manual, from the leadership chapter to the environment of care chapter. It uses elements of performance (EPs) to determine hospitals' compliance with standards. The Joint Commission's 2008 HR standards listed in the following section summarize its expectations for competency (Joint Commission Resources 2008).

Chapter 1

Standard HR.1.20
A staff member's qualifications are consistent with his or her job responsibilities.

This requirement pertains to staff members, students, and volunteers who work in the same capacity as staff members who provide care, treatment, and services. This also includes contract staff members.

It seems simple enough, doesn't it? Steve Doe applies to be an emergency department (ED) staff RN. HR representatives compare what Steve Doe put on his application to the RN job description for an ED staff nurse to determine whether he meets the qualifications for the position. The criteria on the job description state, "Licensed RN in the state of Texas. Minimum of two years recent clinical experience in an ED required. Current card in basic life support for healthcare providers, advanced cardiac life support, and pediatric advanced life support required. Certified emergency nurse preferred." Steve Doe had better meet these requirements.

As we indicated in the Preface, the process for verifying these credentials is of utmost importance to the safety of your patients. Your organization needs a system to ensure that your nurses are who they say they are and have the experience and documentation to back it up. A surveyor may ask an ED nurse (who happens to be Steve Doe), "What is required to work in this department?" The nurse tells the surveyor what was required for his position. The surveyor may then ask for an ED staff RN job description as well as Steve's file to see whether the hospital did indeed verify that all the screening requirements were met and that there is a record indicating that the requirements are still being met.

Standard HR.2.10
The hospital provides initial orientation.

The EPs establish that this standard applies to each staff member, student, and volunteer at your facility. The EPs encompass the following:

- Key elements of orientation that must occur before staff members provide care
- Orientation of the staff to identified key elements prior to providing care
- The hospital's mission and goals

- Organization- and relevant unit-, setting-, or program-specific (e.g., safety and infection control) policies and procedures

- Specific job duties and responsibilities and unit-, setting-, or program-specific job duties related to safety and infection control

- Cultural diversity and sensitivity

- Patient rights and ethical aspects of care, treatment, and services and the process to address ethical issues

In addition, the forensic staff (i.e., police who bring in prisoners) must know how to:

- Interact with patients

- Respond to life safety codes

- Communicate through appropriate channels

- Define their roles in clinical seclusion and restraint

It is expected that, during orientation, the hospital assesses and documents the competency level of the new hire so that by the end of orientation the person is deemed competent (sample orientation competency assessment tools for an RN and nurse assistant appear in Chapter 6). This standard highlights the fact that competence in nursing is not a one-size-fits-all arrangement. Although your ability to synthesize your competency assessment practices across your entire organization will ultimately determine your success, you must be able to customize your tools and process to their intended audience. However, keep in mind that the organization is not expected to shoulder this responsibility alone. Provision 5.2 under the ANA's Code of Ethics states that the nurse "owes the same duties to self as to others, including the responsibility to preserve integrity and safety, to maintain competence, and to continue personal and professional growth" (ANA 2001).

As a result, state BNEs' rules and regulations may dictate competency expectations. These regulations vary, but many discuss competency pertaining to:

- Role delineation for "respondent superiors" (i.e., adult nurse practitioners, licensed practical nurses, licensed vocational nurses, new grads, and unlicensed personnel)

- Scopes of practice for patient care

Chapter 1

- Peer review
- Informed consent
- Medication administration
- Pain management (including epidurals)
- Conscious sedation/analgesia
- Patient/family education
- Blood administration
- Population-specific care

Standard HR.2.20
Staff and licensed independent practitioners, as appropriate, can describe or demonstrate their roles and responsibilities relative to safety.

The EPs for this standard include:

- Risks within the hospital environment
- Actions to eliminate, minimize, and report risks
- Procedures to follow in the event of an adverse event
- Reporting processes for common problems, failures, and user errors

This standard coincides with the introduction of the National Patient Safety Goals (NPSGs) and new requirements by The Joint Commission. The NPSGs are derived from a sentinel event advisory group, and the requirements are generally more prescriptive than other Joint Commission requirements. They are based upon aggregate data following national trends of sentinel patient events. As of January 1, 2005, The Joint Commission began to incorporate NPSGs into the accreditation survey (Joint Commission 2007). The NPSGs highlight the link between competent patient care and safety. To fulfill your hospital's mission of delivering safe patient care, there is significant value in validating healthcare professionals' competencies associated with these goals.

Also note that licensed independent practitioners (LIPs) have been included in HR.2.20. An LIP is someone who is authorized by law and the hospital to "provide care and services without direction or supervision, within the scope of the individual's license and consistent with individually granted clinical privileges" (Joint Commission Resources 2008). LIPs give medical orders for patient care. The individual is credentialed through the hospital medical staff committee.

2008 National Patient Safety Goals

Goal #1. Improve the accuracy of patient identification.

- Use at least two patient identifiers when providing care, treatment, or services

Goal #2. Improve the effectiveness of communication among caregivers.

- For verbal or telephone orders or for telephonic reporting of critical test results, verify the complete order or test result by having the person receiving the information record and "read back" the complete order or test result

- Standardize a list of abbreviations, acronyms, symbols, and dose designations that are not to be used throughout the organization

- Measure and assess, and if appropriate, take action to improve the timeliness of reporting, and the timeliness of receipt by the responsible licensed caregiver, of critical tests and critical results and values

- Implement a standardized approach to "hand off" communications, including an opportunity to ask and respond to questions

Goal #3. Improve the safety of using medications.

Look-alike, sound-alike names for medications and concentrated electrolyte drug concentrations are sentinel events waiting to happen. Studies have been initiated regarding the advent of computer-based medication administration to improve the safety of such medications. For example, bar code scanning, the latest technological advance, may decrease medication errors. But with this new technology comes a new set of competencies. These competencies must be validated before care is initiated with the new technology, and your assessments must be ongoing. In addition, this goal expects you to:

Chapter 1

- Identify and review at least annually look-alike, sound-alike drugs used in the organization
- Label all medications, medication containers (e.g., syringes, medicine cups, and basins) or other solutions on and off the sterile field
- Reduce the likelihood of patient harm associated with anticoagulation therapy

Goals #4–6. Not applicable.

Goal #7. Reduce the risk of healthcare-associated infections.
This includes:

- Compliance with World Health Organization or CDC hand hygiene guidelines
- Managing all cases of unanticipated death or loss of function from a healthcare-associated infection as a sentinel event

OSHA mandates competency in maintaining health requirements for those working in healthcare facilities. These OSHA competencies must be validated. Tuberculosis testing, use of personal protective equipment, use of needless systems, latex allergy requirements, and so on stress the need for those involved in direct patient care to be competent in delivering that care to your patients.

Goal #8. Accurately and completely reconcile medications across the continuum of care.
A process must be developed for obtaining and documenting a complete list of current patient medications—with the involvement of the patient—upon admission. The process includes a comparison of the medications the organization provides to those on the list. This list is communicated to the next provider of service upon transfer or referral within or outside of the organization and is provided to the patient on discharge from the organization. Goal #8 requires interpersonal communication and listening skills, competencies that are challenging but not impossible for your organization to validate.

Goal #9. Reduce the risk of patient harm resulting from falls.
For this goal, the organization must implement a fall reduction program, including an evaluation of the effectiveness of the program. Staff members, patients, and families must be educated on the fall reduction program.

Goals #10–12. Not applicable.

Goal #13. Encourage patients' active involvement in their own care as a patient safety strategy.
The organization must define and communicate the means for patients and their families to report concerns about safety and encourage them to do so. When patients know what to expect, they are more aware of possible errors and choices. Patients can be an important source of information regarding potential adverse events and hazardous conditions.

Goal #14. Not applicable.

Goal #15. The organization identifies safety risks inherent in its client population.

- The organization identifies clients at risk for suicide

Goal #16. Improve recognition and response to changes in a patient's condition. (Note: this requirement has a one-year phase-in period that includes defined expectations for planning, development, and testing ["milestones"] at three, six, and nine months in 2008, with the expectation of full implementation by January 1, 2009.)

- The organization selects a suitable method that enables healthcare staff members to directly request additional assistance from one or more specially trained individuals when the patient's condition appears to be worsening

- Formal education for urgent response policies and practices is conducted with the people who may request assistance and the people who may respond to those requests

Many organizations have implemented Rapid Response Teams to meet this standard. Early response to changes in a patient's condition may reduce cardiopulmonary arrests and patient mortality.

The list of NPSGs will probably lengthen with time. However, using evidence-based practice and benchmarking, facilities with the best-practice data to reduce risk and enhance patient safety will continue to drive competency in practice in the future.

Standard HR.2.30
Ongoing education, including inservices, training, and other activities, maintains and improves competence.

With this standard, The Joint Commission expects that measuring competency at your organization is an ongoing process. In other words, it isn't enough for you to assume that your system for validating competencies at orientation will cover your employees for the length of their employment. EPs for this standard expect:

- Training to occur when job responsibilities and duties change (e.g., when an ED nurse transfers to the neonatal ICU [NICU] but has never worked in a NICU setting).

- That participation in ongoing training will increase staff, student, or volunteer knowledge of work-related issues.

- Ongoing education to be appropriate to the needs of the population(s) served, safety, and infection prevention and control, and to comply with laws and regulations.

- Staff members to know how to manage and report unanticipated events.

- Inservices and staff education to incorporate methods of team training, when appropriate.

- That learning needs to be identified through performance improvement findings and other data analysis. Education is planned, implemented, and evaluated for effectiveness.

- Documentation of ongoing staff education.

Most state boards of nursing mandate continuing education requirements for nurses who apply for relicensure. Hospitals striving for recognition through the ANCC Magnet Recognition Program® are required to foster an environment of continual learning for their nursing staff or risk losing their designation. This standard underlines the need for ongoing education and competency validation at your organization.

Standard HR.3.10
Staff competence to perform job responsibilities is assessed, demonstrated, and maintained.

Once again, this standard stresses that competency assessment be an ongoing process. An EP for this standard may be point-of-care testing (POCT) for the CAP. For example, for CAP accreditation to be maintained, staff members must be competent to perform POCT (CAP Web site). This testing goes beyond knowing how to do a fingerstick test for blood-glucose testing. CAP wants to know who is allowed to do POCT. Are staff members involved in quality control testing and documentation as defined by hospital policy? What tests are allowed to be performed outside of the main hospital laboratory, and what areas are allowed to do what? Examples of POCT that may need to be validated include (but may not be limited to):

- Hemacult
- Urine dipstick
- Nitrazine pH
- Blood glucose

Competency and litigation

Regulatory agencies and legal issues are conjoined in HR.3.10. What is the link? Competency assessment is "systematic and allows for a measurable assessment of the person's ability to perform required activities" (Joint Commission Resources 2008). The EPs do not say that you have to use a certain form or have a certain methodology, but you do have to use a systematic measurable process.

In addition, whoever assesses competency must be qualified to do so. The leadership team must know the qualifications of the staff members caring for the patient population served and is accountable and responsible for maintaining a competent staff. For example, an ED nurse cannot deem another ED nurse competent in managing an overdose patient if the "assessor" has managed only one overdose patient. Peer review is critical to competency assessment, but careful consideration must be given to the process.

Plaintiffs' attorneys in legal cases use expert witnesses to verify issues related to competency. For example, the expert ED nurse called on the case of an overdose patient may manage several overdoses every day. This credible witness likely embodies the standard for excellence and competency in practice. If the patient had a negative outcome following a gastric lavage, the expert may be able to dispute the defendant organization's method used to measure competency of ED staff nurses caring for overdose patients.

Case study
Surveyors tracing for competent care

The staff members at Healthcare Hospital are in their second day of a four-day Joint Commission survey. Wanda, the nurse surveyor, is in the critical-care unit (CCU) focusing on a tracer patient named Mrs. D., who was admitted from the ED. Mrs. D. tried to commit suicide in the ED. She was lavaged for her overdose, intubated, and transferred to the CCU.

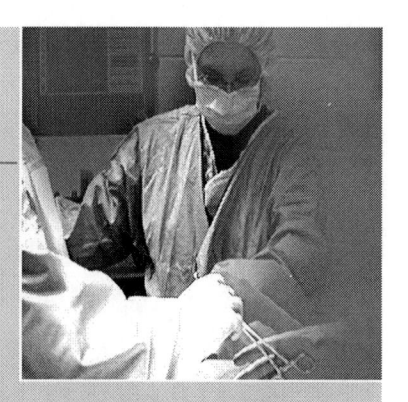

The Joint Commission's tracer methodology strives to ensure that the same standard of care is used throughout the facility by retracing the care delivered to sample patients (or tracers), so Wanda asks the nurse manager to gather three caregivers associated with this patient's case. She also requests that she pull their personnel files because Wanda wants to first ask these nurses various questions regarding the care the patient received and their competency to deliver that care. Then she'll verify whether accreditation standards have been met by reviewing their files. The three employees are:

- A new graduate who is going through a critical-care internship
- An RN with 25 years of experience in critical care
- A certified nursing assistant (CNA) who is a foreign nurse preparing to sit for the boards in the United States

Wanda also wants to review the nurse manager's file to verify that she meets the competency standards required of her as a member of the leadership team at this facility; she wants to know what training she has had to become a leader. Wanda then proceeds to walk around the unit and delves further into the standards for hospital accreditation.

Based upon federal and state regulatory requirements discussed in this chapter, can you think of some of the important questions Wanda will ask the staff, physician, patient (if this vented patient can participate), and family?

Wanda may ask whether the new graduate is competent to take care of a ventilator patient. If so, how was that validated? If she is not competent, what is the action plan? If the nurse with 25 years of experience is her preceptor, how was she deemed competent? Can the CNA, who is a nurse in her country of origin, interpret the monitor strips correctly?

How would Wanda ensure the timely and accurate assessment of competencies for these personnel? Could she pull job descriptions? Performance evaluations? Competency checklists, or skill sheets? Is your organization ready for that?

Your organization must ask itself, "Are the right people taking care of the right patients for the right reasons?" Consider the following:

> **The decline of standards**
> A big-city school system requires a student in the seventh grade to be able to read as well as a fifth grader, who must be able to read as well as a fourth grader, who, in turn, must be able to read as well as a third grader. What's wrong with demanding that a seventh grader be required to read like a seventh grader? How would you like to be operated on by a brain surgeon who graduated from a school that allowed its students to be a year and a half behind in their skills?
> —*Author unknown*

REFERENCES

1. Agnes, M. (Ed). (2006). *Webster's New World College Dictionary*. Cleveland: Wiley Publishing.

2. ANA. (2001). *Code of Ethics for Nurses with Interpretive Statements*. Washington, DC: ANA.

3. ANA. (2007). *Position Statement on Competency*. Silver Springs, MD: ANA.

4. College of American Pathologists. (2007). Available at *www.cap.org*. Accessed November 25, 2007.

5. The Joint Commission. (2007). "A Journey Through the History of The Joint Commission." Available at *www.jointcommission.org/AboutUs/joint_commission_history.htm*. Accessed November 25, 2007.

6. Joint Commission Resources. (2008). *Comprehensive Accreditation Manual for Hospitals: The Official Handbook*. "GL-12." Oakbrook, IL: Joint Commission Resources.

7. Joint Commission Resources. (2008) *Comprehensive Accreditation Manual for Hospitals: The Official Handbook*. "HR2–HR13." Oakbrook, IL: Joint Commission Resources .

8. Joint Commission Resources. (2007). *Comprehensive Accreditation Manual for Hospitals: The Official Handbook*. "Standard NR3.10, *CAMH* Update 1, March 2007, p. NR-4." (Oakbrook, IL: Joint Commission Resources.

9. Joint Commission Resources. (2008). *Comprehensive Accreditation Manual for Hospitals: The Official Handbook*. "Standard NR3.10, *CAMH* Update 1, September 2006, p. HR-12." Oakbrook, IL: Joint Commission Resources.

10. Knight, Tom.(2004). "JCAHO Certification—Dissecting an Institution." *The Nurses' Lounge* September 2004: 26.

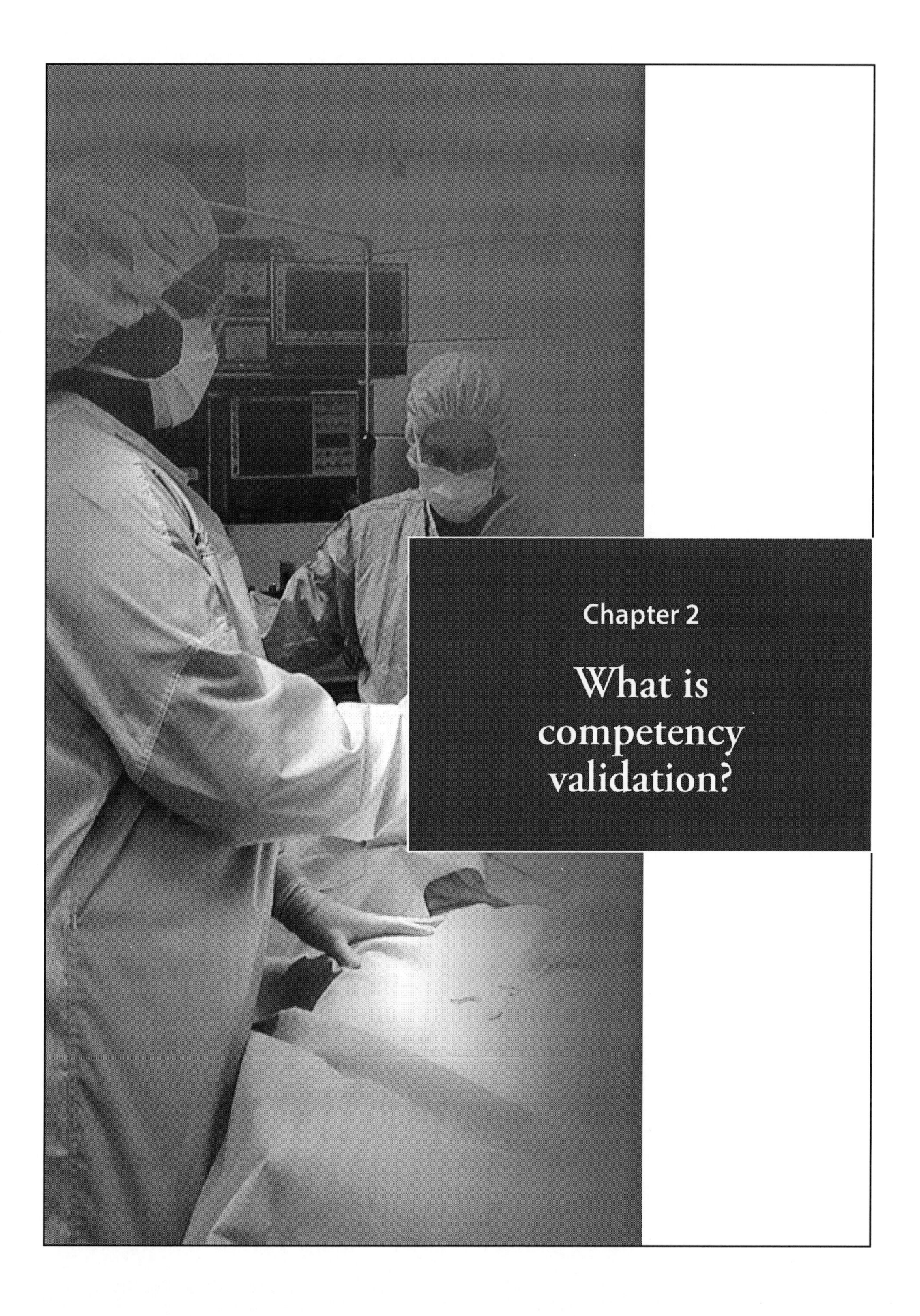

Chapter 2

What is competency validation?

Chapter 2

What is competency validation?

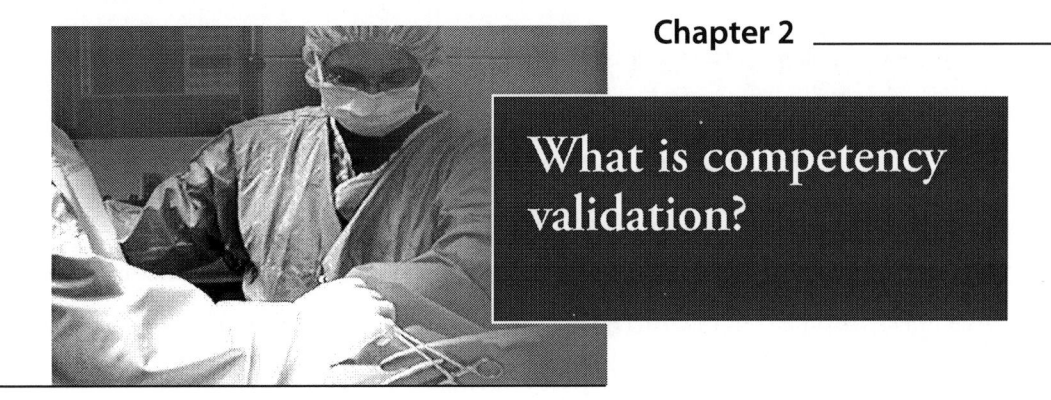

Learning objectives

After reading this chapter, the participant should be able to:

- Identify benefits of competency-based education
- Describe methods of validating competencies

Competency is an issue that affects nursing personnel in all practice settings. Increased pressure from multiple healthcare regulatory agencies and the public necessitates comprehensive evaluation of staff competency. The public demands that nurses demonstrate their competence. This chapter provides information on competency-based education (CBE), as well as on levels and domains of competency. Responsibility for competency validation and the difference between mandatory training and competencies are outlined. The chapter also describes methods for validating competence and options for mapping out or scheduling competencies.

Competency-based education

CBE is one approach commonly used to assess and validate competency. In many ways, CBE reflects a pragmatic concern for doing, not just knowing how to do. Competency models began to evolve during the 1960s as an approach to teacher education, and today CBE models are a widely applied approach to validating competence. In CBE, the learners' self-direction allows educators to act as facilitators to promote learners' goals and is compatible with adults' developmental needs.

Brunt identified that common characteristics of CBE include a learner-centered philosophy, real-life orientation, flexibility, clearly articulated standards, a focus on outcomes, and criterion-reference evaluation methods (Brunt 2007). Most CBE programs focus on outcomes rather than processes.

Generally, CBE programs focus on a specific role and setting and use criteria developed by expert practitioners. CBE emphasizes outcomes in terms of what individuals must know and be able to do and allows flexible pathways for achieving those outcomes. Figure 2.1 provides a comparison of CBE and traditional education.

Figure 2.1

Comparison of CBE and traditional education

Characteristic	CBE programs (Learner-centered)	Traditional education (Teacher-centered)
Basis of instruction	Student outcomes (competencies)	Specific information to be covered
Pace of instruction	Learner sets own pace in meeting objectives	All proceed at pace determined by instructor
How proceed from task to task	Master one task before moving to another	Fixed amount of time on each module
Focus of instruction	Specific tasks included in role	Information that may or may not be part of role
Method of evaluation	Evaluated according to predetermined standards	Relate achievement of learner to other learners

A competency-based approach offers many benefits. These include:

- Having clear guidelines for everyone involved in the process
- Encouraging teamwork
- Enhancing skills and knowledge
- Increasing staff retention
- Reducing staff anxiety
- Improving nursing performance
- Ensuring compliance with the Joint Commission standard that all members of the staff are competent to fulfill their assigned responsibilities

Figure 2.2 provides a sample policy for a competency-based program.

Chapter 2

> **Figure 2.2**
>
> # Sample competency-based program policy
>
> | | |
> |---|---|
> | SUMMA HEALTH SYSTEM HOSPITALS | POLICY: Competency Based Program |
> | AKRON CITY HOSPITAL | SECTION: VI |
> | SAINT THOMAS HOSPITAL | PAGE: 4 |
>
> **PATIENT CARE SERVICES**
> **STAFF POLICY AND PROCEDURE SECTION**
>
> **SUBJECT:**
>
> Summa Health System Hospitals has adopted a competency-based program to ensure that nursing staff are prepared to deliver quality patient care. Assessment of competency begins with orientation and continues throughout employment.
>
> An evaluation of each nursing staff member's competency is conducted at defined intervals throughout the individual's association with the hospital. Performance appraisals may be used as a measure of ongoing competency of nursing employees. Nursing staff members have access to ongoing continuing education programs to enhance their competency.
>
> **DEFINITIONS:**
>
> **Department of Patient Care Services Orientation:** Consists of centralized orientation and unit orientation. Some areas also have a divisional orientation.
>
> - **Centralized Orientation:** Refers to the introduction, reinforcement, and demonstration of general required competencies that a nursing staff member needs to practice within any division of Summa Health System.
>
> - **Divisional Orientation:** Refers to the introduction and application of general practice concepts related to the division assigned. Divisional orientation is reserved for specialties such as critical care, medical-surgical, and operating room.
>
> - **Unit Orientation:** Refers to the clinical application of general and unit-specific competencies for a nursing staff member to practice on his/her assigned unit specialty, or patient population. It also includes geographic and social orientation.

Figure 2.2
Sample competency-based program policy (cont.)

Competency: Skill/activity identified by unit/ division that must be successfully performed to promote quality patient care. Competency is concerned with what the individual can do in the provision of patient care.

- **Departmental Competencies:** Competencies required for all staff assigned to direct patient care, such as BLS.

- **Divisional Competencies:** Selected competencies required within a specific nursing division or specialty, generally included in a curriculum specific to the division, or specialty, such as but not limited to,

    Obstetrics
    - Neonatal resuscitation

    Critical care
    - ACLS
    - EKG interpretation

    Behavioral health
    - Nonviolent crisis intervention

- **Unit-Competencies:** Unit-specific competencies required for nursing staff members working on that unit/specialty patient population.

Competence Assessment Process

Competence assessment for nursing staff and volunteers who are providing direct patient care is based on the following:

1. Populations served, including age ranges and specialties.

2. Competencies required for role and provision of care.

3. Competencies assessed during orientation.

Figure 2.2
Sample competency-based program policy (cont.)

4. Unit specific competencies that need to be assessed or reassessed on a yearly basis, based on care modalities, age ranges, techniques, procedures, technology, equipment, skills needed, or changes in law and regulations.

5. Appropriate assessment methods for the skill being assessed.

6. Delineation of who is qualified to assess competence.

7. Description of action taken when improvement activities lead to a determination that a staff member with performance problems is unable or unwilling to improve.

Ongoing Competence: Refers to periodic assessment of selected competencies for the nursing staff member practicing within a division and on a specific nursing unit; may be centralized or division/unit specific.

Required competency will include:
1. Annual performance appraisal.

2. Completion of mandatory organizational education and other inservices designated as mandatory for personnel.

3. BLS health care provider course or renewal every 2 years (RNs, LPNs, technicians, medical assistants).

4. BLS heartsaver course every 2 years (nursing assistants, unit secretaries).

5. Unit competencies.

Required specialty competencies will include the above as well as unit competencies. Each year unit based competencies will be reviewed by the unit manager and required competencies changed based on individual needs of the unit, identified QI needs or problems identified, changes in patient population, care modalities,

Figure 2.2

Sample competency-based program policy (cont.)

technology, etc. A complete list of chosen unit based competencies will be maintained in staff development.

DIVISIONAL COMPETENCIES (continued):

Assessing Competence

1. Competency checklists will be used to assess demonstrated and ongoing competence. This ensures consistency in evaluating the steps to perform the skill.

2. When introducing new technology or procedures into the clinical area, the initial training is done by individuals with documented experience in that procedure (e.g., physician, nurses from that specialty, vendor representatives, etc.). A core group of staff members or a single individual is trained and confirms competency of other staff members after they personally demonstrate competence in that skill.

3. Ongoing competence will be assessed by an individual with documented competence in that skill. That competence may be determined by their role (e.g., advanced practice nurse, staff development instructor, unit manager, specialty coordinator, etc.), frequency performing the skill, or by already having demonstrated competence in that skill.

Documentation of Competence

1. Each unit will have a Continuing Education Record and Employee Profile binder.

2. Each employee will have an individual record in the binder.

3. It is the responsibility of the individual staff member to complete the education record and employee profile.

4. Preceptors, Unit Managers and Associate Unit Managers can sign employees off on their competencies.

Figure 2.2
Sample competency-based program policy (cont.)

5. Approved list of preceptors by unit will be listed in the front of the binder.

6. All competency checklists specific to each department and division will be located in the front of the education binder.

7. The required competencies are listed on the Continuing Education Record and Employee Profile for department and division.

8. The staff required to complete the competency, activity, or self-learning packets are listed on the profile.

9. RNs are required to complete all competencies, activities or self-learning packets.

10. Competencies are to be completed by December of each year and will be utilized in annual performance appraisal.

11. Once the employee demonstrates competency to preceptor they need to have preceptor sign off on the employee profile.

12. Employees can fax or give this profile to education department to include information on electronic continuing education record (employee needs to submit copy of contact hour certificate).

13. The back of the profile is for staff document continuing education/contact hours, presentations that they have attended.

14. Employees still needed to sign their names that they completed the self-learning packet on sign in sheets.

15. Staff not able to accurately perform any competency will be referred to the Unit Manager. They will be given 30 days to meet this competency and will not be assigned to a patient who requires that competency during that

Figure 2.2
Sample competency-based program policy (cont.)

period. At the end of 30 days if they cannot meet the required competency they will be transferred from that area and reassigned to another area with an open position in which they meet the competencies. Continued failure to demonstrate required competencies leads to a practice plan for improvement and eventual termination.

REFERENCE:

Brunt, B. A. (2007). *Competencies for Staff Educators: Tools to Evaluate and Enhance Nursing Professional Development.* Marblehead, MA: HCPro

---

Mary H. Ward, BSN, MBA, RN, CNAA-BC
Vice President/CNO Patient Care Services

Barbara Brunt, MA, MN, RN-BC
Director, Nursing Education and
Staff Development

Source: Summa Health Systems Hospitals, Akron, OH. Reprinted with permission.

Chapter 2

Defining competencies

Confusion surrounding the competency movement is a result of the numerous definitions used to address this concept, and definitions vary widely. The definition used in this chapter is that *competency* is a broad statement describing an aspect of practice that must be developed and demonstrated, and *competence* is the achievement and integration of many competencies into practice, or the overall ability to perform. Competency is about what people can do. It is the integration of cognitive, affective, and psychomotor domains of practice. It involves both the ability to perform in a given context and the capacity to transfer knowledge and skills to new tasks and situations.

Classifying competencies by domains and levels

Once an institution has a clear definition of competency, the next step is to classify competencies by domains and levels.

Domains of competency

Dorothy del Bueno, a recognized expert in nursing CBE, described three domains of competence—technical, interpersonal, and critical thinking skills—that are often addressed in literature. Del Bueno developed a performance-based development system (PBDS) that focuses on these three aspects of practice.

The PBDS provides initial assessment data about a nurse's ability to perform and identifies learning needs. Clinical judgment skills are assessed through a series of videotaped patient scenarios in which the nurse must identify the problem and outline what steps should be taken to solve that problem to assess his or her ability to recognize and manage patient problems and give rationale for interventions taken.

Patient kardexes and care plans also provide the opportunity to assess the nurse's ability to prioritize scheduled activities for patients, and event cards are used to assess the nurse's ability to determine the priority for unscheduled events. If a task is a must-do event, the nurse must identify the appropriate action to be taken.

Audiotapes of various nurse–physician or nurse–nurse interactions assess the nurse's ability to recognize ineffective interpersonal strategies and identify interventions that could achieve more desirable outcomes. Some technical skills are demonstrated in a clinical laboratory setting, whereas others are demonstrated on the clinical unit. After the nurse completes the assessment, the assigned clinical instructor completes a profile documenting the assessment, develops an action plan that summarizes the findings, and identifies learning needs. The focus on technical skills, interpersonal skills, and critical-thinking skills is helpful, although the initial evaluation of competence for new hires may be too time-intensive.

Some roles may require competencies in other domains appropriate for those roles. For instance, managers must demonstrate leadership competencies. In our increasingly diverse healthcare environment, it is important for staff members to demonstrate cultural competence when caring for patients of different backgrounds. Cultural competence encompasses not only racial diversity, but also diversity in age, culture, religious beliefs, sexual orientation, and other demographic factors. Cultural competence builds first on an awareness of one's own cultural perspective and then acknowledges the perspectives of another culture on the same issue.

Levels of competency

People function at various levels, and it is important to identify those differences in competencies. Pat Benner, a nurse theorist, differentiated five levels of skill acquisition in her novice-to-expert theory: novice, advanced beginner, competent, proficient, and expert. This book classifies competencies into three levels: beginner, intermediate, and expert.

Levels of performance are often differentiated by the ability to analyze and synthesize information. Beginners have limited exposure to the tasks expected of them and function at a basic level. With time and the development of expertise, they acquire more skills and can identify potential problems and act accordingly—and they reach the intermediate level. Experts have a wealth of knowledge to draw upon and frequently anticipate problems and plan strategies to avoid them.

A competency on performing a respiratory assessment would be a beginning competency for an RN, whereas initiating actions to prevent or minimize complications based on one's assessment data would be an intermediate competency, and appropriately responding to subtle changes in respiratory assessment data would be a more expert competency.

Chapter 2

Who performs competency validation?

After identifying expected competencies for each job classification, the next step is to determine who can validate competencies. This role will vary depending on the resources and types of personnel in the facility.

The American Nurses Association's *Nursing: Scope and Standards of Practice* addresses the mandate that nurses must provide care competently and keep up with current nursing practice (ANA 2004). Individuals at all levels of the organization must assume personal responsibility to maintain their competence and ensure that they follow the system established by their organization to validate their competence.

Every organization has a responsibility to ensure that all staff members who provide patient care are educated appropriately and are competent to fulfill their job responsibilities and meet acceptable standards. To meet the requirements of The Joint Commission and other accrediting bodies, organizations must also ensure ongoing competence of employees (Joint Commission Resources 2008). To do this, they must establish a competency system and determine who can validate competence.

Various individuals or groups with documented expertise in an area can validate competence of others. For instance, an agency could determine that either RNs or licensed practical nurses (LPNs) can validate nursing assistants' (NAs') competency in taking vital signs. For lifting and transfer techniques, someone from physical therapy or nurses could validate competency. For some skills, someone in one job category could validate the competence of another person in that same category. For instance, an RN experienced in critical care could validate the competence of a fellow RN in measuring cardiac output.

Organizations must identify clearly who can validate competencies and ensure that they have the appropriate education, experience, or expertise with that skill to perform the competency validation. Anyone who validates competence should be trained to do so (see Chapter 4) and should use an established competency checklist to ensure consistency with the evaluation process (see Chapter 6).

Mandatory training versus competencies

There is often confusion between competencies and mandatory training required by regulatory agencies or institutional policy. Most organizations require that all staff members review a variety of safety topics on a

What is competency validation?

yearly basis, such as fire safety, dealing with emergency situations (e.g., cardiac arrests, disasters, hazardous materials, etc.), and cultural diversity. Institutions have a variety of ways to achieve this task. Some distribute self-learning packets (SLPs) containing the essential information and require everyone to review that material annually. Some SLPs may require that the individual take a posttest, and others may require simply that the individual read the information. Institutions that have computer capabilities may require personnel to complete safety programs online. Some may hold face-to-face sessions, which may or may not include some hands-on practice with the skill, for reviewing the information.

The difference between mandatory training and competency validation is that the latter requires demonstration of the skill, whereas the former does not necessarily do so. To further clarify the difference, the following list outlines some of the common safety topics required by regulatory agencies:

- Cultural competence and ethical conduct
- Privacy and confidentiality issues (e.g., Health Insurance Portability and Accountability Act of 1996 [HIPAA] requirements)
- Fire safety
- Disaster preparedness
- Emergency codes
- Electrical safety
- Infection control and bloodborne pathogens
- Institutional safety plan and patient safety
- Back safety
- Emergency response to various threats (e.g., bombs, patient/family violence)

An example of competency is many organizations' requirement that personnel maintain competence in basic life support (BLS), which requires a staff member to complete appropriate courses as a healthcare provider, heart saver, or advanced cardiac life-support provider.

The focus on competencies is on what the individual can do, not what he or she knows, and competencies must be measured in a simulated or clinical setting. One example of a competency that can be demonstrated without specific patient contact is blood-glucose testing. Any healthcare provider who tests blood sugar results must get an accurate reading because treatment is based on those results. The lab can provide a contrast material to the units so that individuals can run a sample and send their results to the lab. The lab can determine the accuracy of the individual's reading and his or her ability to use the machine correctly by comparing the individual's results with the test material.

Mapping competencies for orientation, annual assessments

You can determine which skills should be evaluated each year in a variety of ways. Selected competencies can be based on the needs of an individual unit, identified quality-improvement needs or problems, changes in patient population, care modalities, or new technologies. Summarized performance appraisal results could be used to indicate the particular competencies staff members need to develop further. Skills that are not used frequently but that present high risk to the patient can also be validated. Most institutions require some safety training annually, as well as BLS courses; these can also be part of the competency process. Many organizations are working toward integrating their performance appraisal and competency management systems. We will discuss this further in Chapter 3.

Some institutions focus on skills that are high-risk, low-volume, or problem-prone (Cooper 2002).

High-risk activities can cause serious (or deadly) damage to a patient or staff member if performed incorrectly. Look at high-risk activities closely. If they are performed every day, they are considered high-volume. High-volume activities do not necessarily need to be reviewed every year, although they should be a part of your orientation program. The assumption is that you perform the activity so often that you know it well.

Low-volume skills are not performed very often within your department, but employees still need to know how to perform them well. These skills should be reviewed at least annually. If an activity is both high-risk and low-volume, you definitely should include it in your annual review.

Problem-prone skills are the subject of unusual occurrence reports or other error reporting forms or quality assurance data. These data should be reviewed regularly, because they are an excellent source of skill or knowledge deficits that become annual competencies. Near misses are also serious enough for a review.

Elizabeth Parsons and Mary Bona Capka suggested a model to determine how frequently skills should be assessed based on risk (Parsons and Capka 1997). Although this may be more detailed than necessary for some organizations, it may be helpful to identify high-risk procedures. The following are the key factors in their model:

- **Incident frequency:** This is determined by a rating scale that includes occurrence, quality improvement, and compliance data. Occurrence scores are ranked on a Likert-type scale (e.g., 5 = daily; 4 = once per week; 3 = once per month; 2 = once in six months; 1 = once per year or less; 0 = never). Incidents are defined as untoward incidents, equipment problems, staff noncompliance, or infection control data reported in the past 12 months. The more incidents, the higher the score.

- **Use/performance frequency:** This identifies the equipment use or competency performance. It uses the same Likert-type scale as the incident frequency scale, but with reversed scoring (e.g., 5 = once per year or less; 1 = daily). If procedures are performed infrequently, important steps may be inadvertently omitted. The more frequently the staff member performs the competency, the lower the score.

- **Patient/operator risk:** This scale scores each item according to the risk to the patient or operator if the competency is performed incorrectly. The highest score (i.e., 5 = operator or patient death) is assigned to competencies for which there is great risk to the patient or staff member, where the lowest score (i.e., 1 = barely any risk) is used if there is no significant risk to the patient or staff member.

- **Skill complexity:** This score captures the skills' complexity and is based on Benner's novice-to-expert model. Skills that the new graduate should be able to perform without supervision would rank lowest (1 or 2), whereas skills that require application of theoretical principles in creative and innovative ways score highest (9 or 10). In this manner, skills necessary to perform an identified competency factor into decisions made about the frequency of assessment.

The formula that Parsons and Capka used captured all these components, with risk being identified as the most crucial factor. Additional weight or value was given to the patient/operator risk score. Their formula appears in the box that follows. Scores range from 0 to 100.

> Incident frequency (I) + user frequency (U) + skill complexity (C)
> X patient/operator risk (R) = Total score (T), or
> (I + F + C) R = T

Chapter 2

For example, a skill such as providing immediate support for a cardiac arrest (e.g., BLS or advanced life support) would have a relatively high risk score. The incident frequency would encompass the number of untoward events during codes in the past year (in this case, 1). User frequency would vary, but for most non-critical-care areas, it would be rated high (a rating of 5) because it is not routinely performed in those areas. Complexity would be rather high (a rating of 8) because a code is a complex patient-care situation, and the risk would be high (a rating of 5) because inappropriate performance of the competency could lead to patient death. A potential score of 70 could be obtained using the formula given earlier: (1 + 5 + 8) 5 = 70.

Your method for mapping competencies to be validated needs to be flexible enough to allow for changes or modifications based on environmental factors. For instance, a new piece of equipment might require the staff to demonstrate competency in using that equipment. The system would need to be flexible enough to include that as an additional competency in a timely manner for the affected staff members.

Methods for validating competencies

It is important to realize that there are numerous ways to validate competencies. One of the most common methods is the skills checklist, which is described in Chapter 6. However, there are many other ways that competence can be validated (Avillion, Brunt, and Ferrell 2007).

Posttests

Posttests are one method for documenting cognitive knowledge and are sometimes used as a method for documenting competence. However, when competency is defined as the overall ability to perform, many tests do not have a performance aspect. One way that tests can be used is to document basic knowledge so that participants don't have to take a course or program when they can show that they have the basic knowledge required in that course. For instance, someone with critical-care experience could take a posttest to document that he or she has sufficient knowledge about a particular skill (e.g., cardiac monitoring) and, as a result, does not have to take that session of the curriculum. However, this would not take the place of validating his or her skills in the clinical area. Some tests may provide a written description, a videotape or audiotape, a live simulation, or printed or projected still pictures, and then present specific questions to which the test taker must respond. Del Bueno's PBDS uses this approach to validate competency.

Observations of daily work

Observations of daily work, such as patient rounds or medical-record reviews, can be a means of validating competency. Specific interactions or skills can be directly observed as someone performs his or her work, and patient outcomes/documentation can be observed as well. This provides an opportunity for multiple observations and addresses one of the problems with checklists, which usually gather data from only one observation of a task. When staff members know they are being observed, they have a tendency to go through all the steps correctly when they might not normally do so.

Case studies

Case studies are another means of validating competency. Individuals can describe how they would provide care for a particular patient or how they would deal with a particular scenario presented to them. These can also be used to address age-specific competencies. After someone describes how he or she would take care of a 37-year-old diabetic patient, the assessor could ask that person what he or she would do differently if the patient was 65 years old. The person's description of the factors he or she would consider and how he or she would alter the patient's care could be used to document the person's ability to care for patients of different ages.

Peer review/360° evaluation

Peer review, or a technique called "360° evaluation," is another method for validating competency. The 360° evaluation incorporates feedback from as many people who interact with a staff member as is feasible. For an RN, these people might include peers, LPNs, NAs, representatives of other disciplines, and the RN's manager. The use of different sources of information and different measures to evaluate competence increases validity.

Exemplars

Exemplars are narrative descriptions of practice. Individuals describe how they handled a particular situation, in essence writing or telling a story about it. Their narrative allows the clinician to describe the step-by-step progression of the incident, as well as the feelings, thoughts, and conclusions from their reflection of the situation. These exemplars can be part of portfolios that can provide concrete examples of competence in a particular area.

Simulated events

Simulated events, such as mock codes, can also be used to validate competency. For example, the instructor can use a mannequin in a bed to describe scenarios and ask the participants to respond appropriately. This provides an opportunity for practice and demonstration of skills in a nonthreatening environment. Another example is the use of volunteers as simulated patients for staff members to perform assessments or demonstrate various noninvasive skills. Also available are various simulators that provide a realistic environment for demonstration of skills, but these can be costly.

Quality-improvement monitors

Quality-improvement monitors, if they reflect individual performance, are another method for validating competency. These are often related to quality-of-care issues such as falls, documentation, healthcare-acquired infections, and so on. With the ongoing emphasis on performance improvement and quality, most organizations have a quality-improvement program and quality monitors in place. For example, an institution may document compliance with the new HIPAA security requirements by having individuals without name tags approach staff members and tell them that they work for IT services. They may ask the employees for their passwords to check the computer system or tell a secretary they are responding to a call about a computer problem and remove a piece of computer equipment from that secretary's manager's office. If the employee does not follow the established policy, feedback and follow-up are provided.

Scheduling and organizing the competencies

Once the competencies to be validated are determined, the organization needs to communicate them to all staff members and provide the tools necessary to validate those skills. This can be done in a variety of ways. Access to the various checklists or methods to validate competencies should be available for all staff members to use during the validation process.

Some organizations may choose to have competency notebooks on each unit that include a tracking sheet of employees and a list of which competencies need validation for each level of personnel. Samples of skills checklists or other methods to validate competencies should also be included in the notebook. If a computer-tracking system is in place, this can be used to map individual- or role-specific competencies. Then the person who performs the validation could enter that information directly into the computer system.

Some organizations may choose to put the responsibility on individuals to make sure they are validated on the required competencies annually. In this case, the individual healthcare worker is responsible for having the appropriate person validate the skill and would be responsible for ensuring that the appropriate documentation was completed. These data can then be used in the individual's performance appraisal.

Some institutions may schedule various competencies to be completed by everyone in a designated time frame (e.g., during the first quarter, or two months before their annual performance appraisal). Others may allow competency validation to be done anytime during the year, as long as it is completed by a designated deadline. Whatever system the organization uses to ensure that competence is validated must be communicated to all staff members, and a mechanism needs to be put in place to ensure that the process is followed.

A final step in the competency validation process is to set up a mechanism for ongoing review and evaluation of the process. Specific questions to be included in an evaluation of a competence assessment system are provided in Chapter 6.

REFERENCES

1. American Nurses Association. (2004). *Nursing: Scope and Standards of Practice.* Washington, DC: ANA.

2. Avillion, Brunt B., and Ferrell M. 2007. *Nursing Professional Development Review and Resource Manual.* Silver Spring, MD: Institute for Credentialing Innovation.

3. Brunt, Barbara A. (2007). *Competencies for Staff Educators: Tools to Evaluate and Enhance Nursing Professional Development.* Marblehead, MA: HCPro, Inc.

4. Cooper, D. (2002). "The 'C' Word: Competency" in Kristen L. O'Shea, *Staff Development Nursing Secrets.* Philadelphia: Hanley & Belfus.

5. Joint Commission Resources. (2008). *Comprehensive Accreditation Manual for Hospitals: The Official Handbook.* Oakbrook Terrace, IL: Joint Commission Resources.

6. Parsons, Elizabeth C., and Mary Bona Capka. (1997.) "Building a successful risk-based competency assessment model." *AORN Journal* 66(6): 1065–1071.

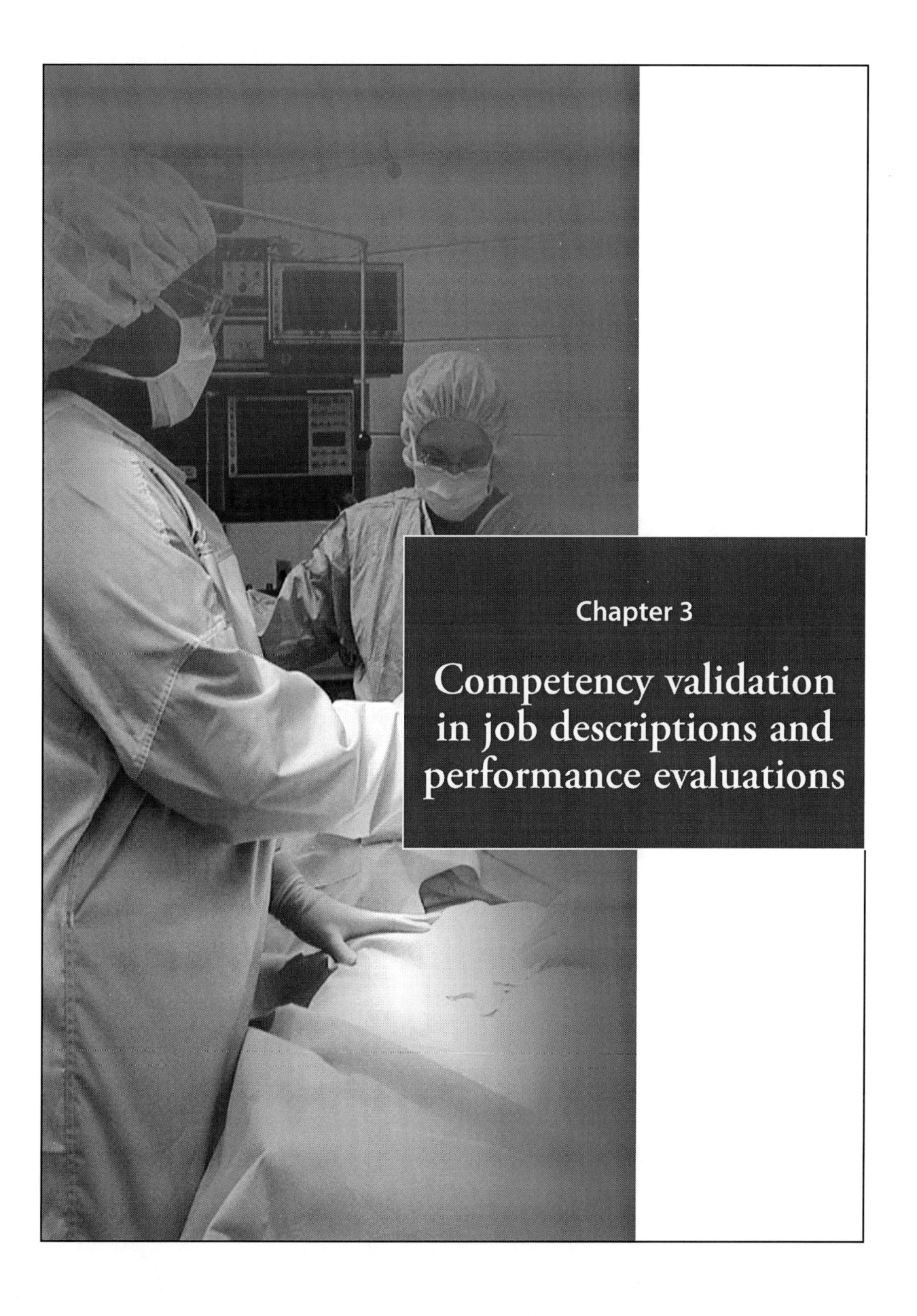

Chapter 3

Competency validation in job descriptions and performance evaluations

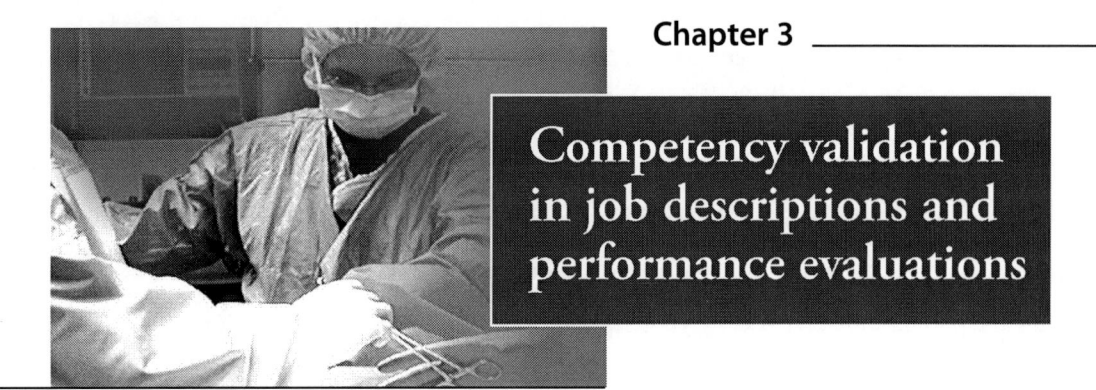

Chapter 3

Competency validation in job descriptions and performance evaluations

Learning objectives

After reading this chapter, the participant should be able to:

- Recognize the benefits of incorporating competency assessment into job descriptions and performance evaluation tools
- Discuss the key elements required of performance-based job descriptions

New technology, legislation, and accreditation standards are changing the job responsibilities of those employed at your organization almost every day. In some cases, these forces make it necessary for your organization to create entirely new job positions to keep pace and ensure safe, quality care. As a result, it is more difficult for hospitals to work with HR to keep job descriptions current, create effective and realistic performance evaluations that are in sync with those job descriptions, and include these tools in a process for assessing initial and ongoing competencies.

In this chapter, we will provide further support for the underpinning theme throughout this book: manageability. That is, not only should you make your competency validation and assessment process compliant and effective, but you should also make it manageable. This chapter discusses the elements required to build competency-based job descriptions.

Competency-based (sometimes called performance-based) job descriptions state employee responsibilities in terms of practice standards, or how these responsibilities must be demonstrated, rather than simply listing

Chapter 3

duties and responsibilities. Competency-based job descriptions, which can double as performance evaluation tools, will also help you meet HR standards set by The Joint Commission.

Although these tools will take a good deal of time to develop, they will help your organization have a more streamlined system for developing performance criteria for your competency validation skill sheets, for assessing age/population-specific competencies, and for tying those assessments into timely performance evaluations. In this chapter, we will discuss:

- The benefits of incorporating competency assessment into your job descriptions and performance evaluation tools
- What The Joint Commission expects from hospitals in this area
- The key elements required of performance-based job descriptions
- Practical tips for complying with The Joint Commission's challenging HR.3.20 standard, which expects timely completion of performance evaluations

The benefits

Your organization can expect several benefits from incorporating competency assessment into its job descriptions and performance evaluations, including the following:

- **Improved efficiency:** As long as you are willing to put the time and effort into building competency-based HR tools, your reward will be a more streamlined, compliant competency assessment process. The performance criteria in your job descriptions can serve as the foundation for your competency validation tools (e.g., skill sheets) and performance evaluations.

- **Improved patient safety:** Defining employees' job responsibilities by widely accepted standards or scopes of practice and holding employees to them will help your organization ensure that patient care is delivered in the safest way possible.

- **Improved employee satisfaction:** Employees need validation from their managers or supervisors about their job performance. They need to know what expectations they have or have not met. Well-developed HR tools composed of measurable performance criteria will make it easier for employees to receive this type of validation.

The Joint Commission's expectations

According to The Joint Commission, one of its competency assessment requirements, HR standard 3.10 (formerly HR5), ranks as the most-cited issue for hospitals accredited by The Joint Commission. HR.3.10 expects that hospitals assess staff competencies in relation to performance expectations outlined in their job descriptions (Joint Commission Resources 2008).

If experience is any measure, it's no wonder organizations struggle with developing effective, time-tested competency assessment tools. In the past, a survey team would visit a facility and make recommendations on how it could improve its competency assessment process or the tools associated with it. The facility would implement modifications based on those recommendations; then, three years later, a different survey team would come in and tell the organization something completely different. As a result, facilities had many different ideas about how to build an effective competency assessment program.

Scenarios such as this one fostered the need for a process, mechanism, or tool to help hospitals develop strong competency assessment programs. A well-developed competency-based job description accomplishes this.

We discussed The Joint Commission's expectations for competency assessment in Chapter 1. As you may recall, the HR.3.10 standard requires that your competency assessment process for staff members, students, and volunteers who work in the same capacity as staff members "providing care, treatment, and services" be based on, above all, populations served and the defined competencies required for each staff member. Therefore, there must be an effort to identify and validate population-specific competencies (which we will discuss in more detail in Chapter 4). Do all healthcare professionals at your facility need to have these competencies validated? No. The Joint Commission specifies that only staff members who provide care, treatment, and services will need to have this done. Your housekeeping staff, for instance, does not need to have population-specific competencies validated.

However, keep in mind that some clinical staff members who aren't licensed will need to have their competencies validated. Pharmacy technicians, for example, are not licensed in many states, yet they fall into the category of clinical staff and deal a lot with medications. Although they're not licensed, pharmacy technicians clearly need to have an understanding of population-specific concerns regarding medication. Dietary aides are another example. They are unlicensed staff members who do not assess or treat patients, but how

Chapter 3

they deliver food differs based on the type of patient. They may need to have population-specific competencies validated.

The Joint Commission also requires you to define a time frame for how often competency assessments are performed and (in HR.3.20) how often performance evaluations are performed. The Joint Commission says this should be done at least once in the three-year accreditation cycle. Most important, however, is that you meet the objectives and goals associated with the time frame your organization chooses. If you fail to meet your expectations, The Joint Commission will cite you.

This highlights the efficiency and effectiveness of a competency assessment process that incorporates both your job descriptions, which spell out the expectations, accountabilities, and competencies associated with the job, and performance evaluations, which allow managers to provide feedback on a regular basis and track employees' progress toward those expectations, accountabilities, and competencies.

Key elements of a competency-based job description

What makes a job description competency- or performance-based?

The foundation for each employee's job description should be the position's qualifications, duties, and responsibilities. However, well-developed competency- or performance-based job descriptions at your facility must state employee responsibilities (i.e., essential functions and nonessential functions) in terms of expected practice standards—in other words, how the responsibilities must be demonstrated. Created by the department manager and understood by the HR department, these standards must have measurable, objective outcomes associated with them. The problem with many job descriptions is that they are written in a way that leads to subjective interpretations by supervisors.

Include an associated rating scale, which includes definitions that have been agreed upon across departments. This scale must be clear and easy to understand for everyone using it. Also include within job descriptions an area for a supervisor to document in narrative format how the employee met expectations.

All the examples in the following section will be based on the job description of a floating RN, in the medical-surgical unit.

Essential and nonessential functions

Essential functions are those tasks, duties, and responsibilities that compose the context of the job (i.e., the means of accomplishing the job's purpose and objectives). The essential functions should be measurable statements that cover the major components of the job for which the person will be held accountable. Figure 3.1 shows an example of two essential functions and their expected performance criteria.

Functions listed as nonessential aren't unimportant—they just are not critical for the performance of the job position. They should be listed as specifically as possible and also should include performance criteria.

Chapter 3

Figure 3.1

Essential functions

1. Assesses and diagnoses patient and family needs to provide quality care to assigned patients.

Performs admission assessment within eight hours of admission or in accordance with specific unit standards.

❑ Consistently does not meet standards	❑ Developmental/ Needs improvement	❑ Consistently meets/ sometimes exceeds standards	❑ Consistently exceeds standards

Identifies and documents nursing diagnosis on patients' plan of care within eight hours of admission.

❑ Consistently does not meet standards	❑ Developmental/ Needs improvement	❑ Consistently meets/ sometimes exceeds standards	❑ Consistently exceeds standards

Identifies and documents patient/family/significant other of admission.

❑ Consistently does not meet standards	❑ Developmental/ Needs improvement	❑ Consistently meets/ sometimes exceeds standards	❑ Consistently exceeds standards

Overall rating

❑ **Consistently does not meet standards**	❑ **Developmental/ Needs improvement**	❑ **Consistently meets/sometimes exceeds standards**	❑ **Consistently exceeds standards**

Performance narrative

2. Develops, discusses, and communicates a realistic problem list (plan of care) for each patient, in collaboration with each patient/family/significant other in order to address all identified needs.

Plan of care will include nursing diagnosis statement for each identified problem.

❑ Consistently does not meet standards	❑ Developmental/ Needs improvement	❑ Consistently meets/ sometimes exceeds standards	❑ Consistently exceeds standards

Develops patient/family/significant other teaching and discharge plan as per unit standard.

❑ Consistently does not meet standards	❑ Developmental/ Needs improvement	❑ Consistently meets/ sometimes exceeds standards	❑ Consistently exceeds standards

Overall rating

❑ **Consistently does not meet standards**	❑ **Developmental/ Needs improvement**	❑ **Consistently meets/sometimes exceeds standards**	❑ **Consistently exceeds standards**

Performance narrative

Organizational competencies

Job descriptions should also include organizational competencies—those that are expected across all departments of the organization for every employee. This will often require you to incorporate competency-based performance standards in sections devoted to (but not limited to):

- Service
- Teamwork
- Communication
- Respect for others
- Time and priority management
- Mandatory safety requirements
- Leadership competencies

Rating scale and definitions

The rating-scale portion of your job descriptions is extremely important. To develop a rating scale that is agreed upon across the organization, consider:

- How many levels of ratings are required to differentiate performance
- How many standards can be identified, maintained, and discriminated in your performance appraisal process
- The reliability of raters across the organization in judging standards
- Whether the rating scale produces improved performance and communication

An example of a rating scale and definitions appears in Figure 3.2.

Figure 3.2

Rating scale and definitions

Consistently exceeds standards	Performance consistently surpasses all established standards. Activities often contribute to improved innovative work practices. This category is to be used for truly outstanding performance.
Consistently meets/ Sometimes exceeds standards	Performance meets all established standards and sometimes exceeds them. Activities contribute to increased unit/departmental results. Employees consistently complete the work that is required and at times go beyond expectations.
Developmental/Needs improvement	Performance meets most but not all established standards. Activities sometimes contribute to unit/department results. This category is to be used for employees who must demonstrate improvement or more consistent performance and/or for employees still learning their job.
Consistently does not meet standards	Performance is consistently below requirements/expectations. Immediate improvement is necessary.

Performance narratives

Performance narratives offer supervisors an opportunity to document their ongoing feedback and evaluation of staff performance. Your goal should be to establish consistency in rating performance across the organization. There is a lot of disagreement regarding what constitutes a good performance evaluation. However, the general thinking is that if you stick to criteria established in your job descriptions you will make it easier on employees and satisfy Joint Commission surveyors.

To this end, a narrative box can be placed at the end of each essential function in your job description (refer back to Figure 3.1). This differs from most traditional performance evaluations, which have space only at the end of the form to document a narrative. This format would allow a supervisor to apply more specific feedback and recommendations.

Compliance tips for HR.3.20

Timely completion of performance evaluations is critical to the success of your entire organization and your Joint Commission survey. To ensure that success, some organizations have established 30- to 90-day windows from the time the reviews are sent out to the time they are due for managers to get the work done. Here is some more advice from industry experts to reduce your turnaround time and reduce your risk of noncompliance with The Joint Commission's HR.3.20:

1. Keep your performance evaluations realistic. A lot of organizations go to great lengths to design comprehensive performance evaluations that address every potential aspect of competency, but managers can't complete them because they are too complicated, says Bud Pate, REHS, practice director for clinical operations improvement for The Greeley Company, a division of HCPro, Inc., in Marblehead, MA.

2. Post reminders. The key to success is discipline, according to Glenn D. Krasker, MHSA, president of Critical Management Solutions, a consulting firm that specializes in medical error risk reduction, in Wilmington, DE. It's best if evaluations are due on employee anniversary dates, rather than all of the organization's evaluations being due on the same date, so the workload is spread out over 12 months.

3. Institute self-evaluations. Help to reduce the burden on supervisors by getting employees to complete a self-assessment of their job performance prior to the performance evaluation, which the manager will amend before it is sent to HR, says Katherine Chamberlain, CPHQ, a consultant in Gloucester, MA.

4. Hold supervisors accountable. Tie in supervisors' evaluations and pay increases to the timelines of their completion of staff evaluations, suggests Krasker.

5. Condense your evaluations. Make sure your evaluations are not overly burdensome. Try to keep the document to one or two pages, says Pate.

6. Automate the process. Online performance evaluation tools help to streamline the process because the forms are easily accessible to everyone and can be filled out quickly and legibly, says Deb Ankowicz, RN, BSN, CPHQ, director of risk management for the University of Wisconsin Hospitals & Clinics, in Madison.

7. Have a blitz day. If managers are running behind schedule, reserve a conference room where they can work without interruptions to get their evaluations done, says Krasker.

Source: Adapted from **Briefings on The Joint Commission newsletter,** *published by HCPro, Inc.*

The key to successfully incorporating your competency assessment process into the ongoing maintenance of job descriptions and the completion of performance evaluations is to develop manageable tools. At the very least, these tools need to identify measurable performance criteria and promote consistent, agreed-upon methods for evaluating the staff (based in part on the populations with which they work) and getting it all done in a timely manner.

REFERENCES

1. Joint Commission Resources. (2008). *Comprehensive Accreditation Manual for Hospitals: The Official Handbook*. Oakbrook Terrace, IL: Joint Commission Resources.

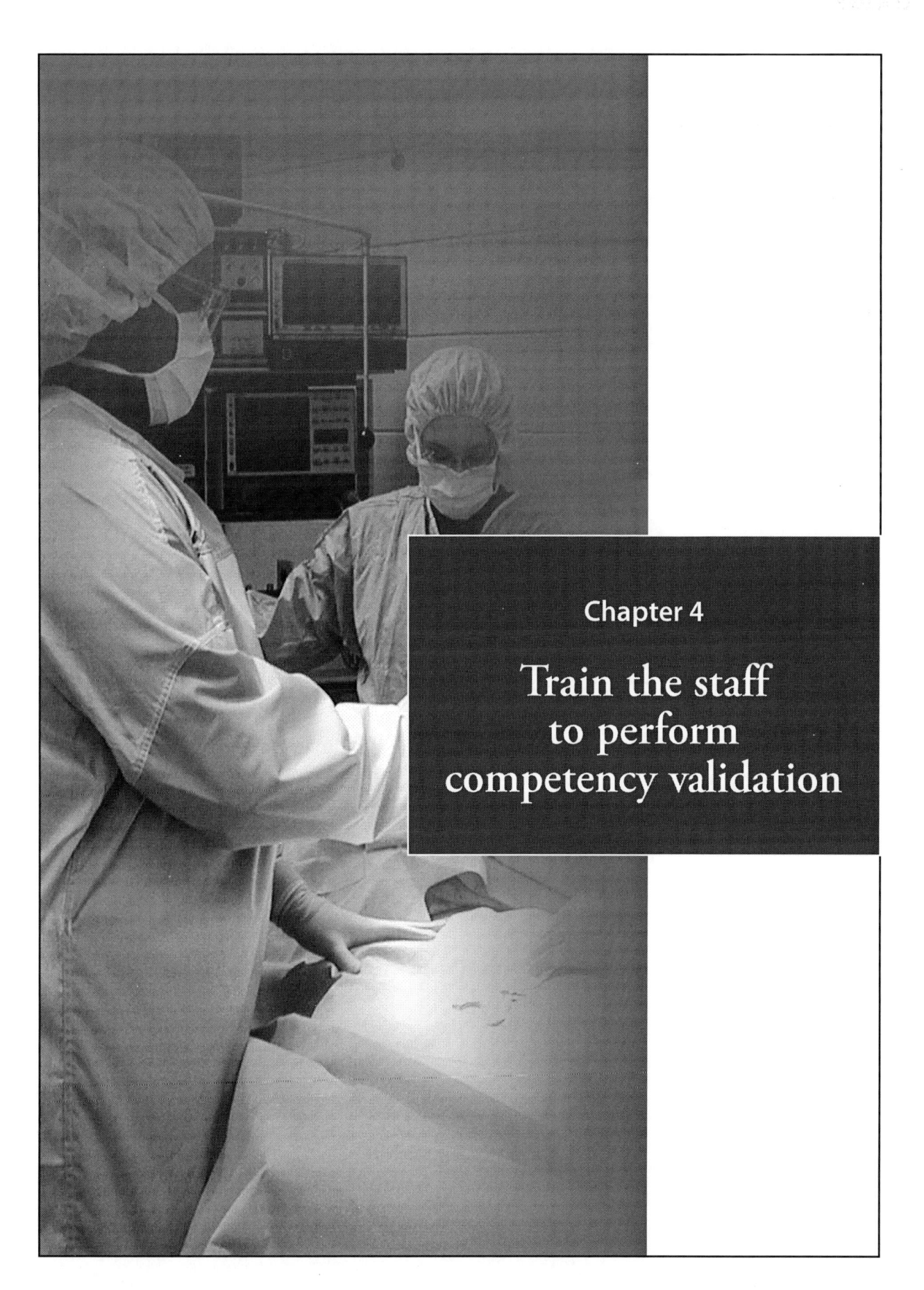

Chapter 4

Train the staff to perform competency validation

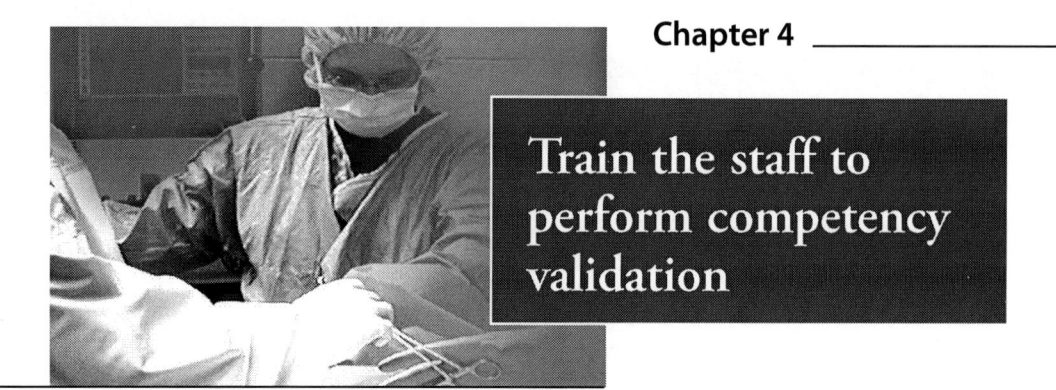

Chapter 4

Train the staff to perform competency validation

Learning objectives

After reading this chapter, the participant should be able to:

- Develop a training program to train staff to perform competency assessment
- Maintain consistency in a competency validation system
- Identify steps for effective program documentation
- Recognize the essential qualities needed by competency assessors

Who performs competency validation within your organization? How are they trained to perform this important responsibility? Ideally, those who assess the competency of others are selected based on their clinical skills and ability to help colleagues enhance job performance. This means they also possess tact and good teaching skills and receive appropriate training prior to evaluating colleagues' job performance. The opposite of this ideal situation is to have all staff members assess the competency of others with little or no training, regardless of their teaching skills.

The truth is, most organizations fall somewhere between these two extremes. The purpose of this chapter is to help you design a practical training program for those staff members responsible for assessing the competency of others.

Chapter 4

Developing a competency assessment training program

Who should be trained to perform competency assessment? First, understand that not all staff members should be trained to assess their colleagues' competency. Competency assessment is an acquired skill that not all healthcare professionals possess.

What qualifications should a competency assessor possess?

- Excellent performance of the competencies being evaluated
- Tact and the desire to help colleagues improve their job performance
- The desire to acquire/enhance adult education skills
- Demonstration of excellent interpersonal communication skills

Now that you know who should be trained, what should you include in the training program? The following components should be part of your competency assessment training and education program.

Purpose

Learners need to understand the purpose and importance of a competency assessment program. You need to be able to demonstrate how job performance is enhanced and patient care improved by adhering to competency criteria. Use quality improvement and risk management data to prove your point. Learners must also understand that The Joint Commission and other accrediting agencies expect staff members to demonstrate their competence, that such competence is evaluated on an ongoing basis, and that each staff member's competence is documented.

Principles of adult learning

Any education program that involves training adults to teach/coach other adults must include an overview of the principles of adult learning (Avillion, Brunt, and Ferrell 2007).

- **Adults must have a valid reason for learning.** Adults want proof that there is a need for learning (i.e., they want to know why it is important for them to participate in an educational activity). For example, suppose the ability to draw arterial blood gases is a competency for all RNs on the medical ICU. Some of them complain that they perform this task frequently and they don't need someone observing them to validate their competency. If you are able to cite quality improvement data indicating a negative trend (e.g., infections, bruising, etc.) due to questionable techniques, you can show them why there is a need for continual competency assessment. National data can also be cited to illustrate the need for keeping "on top" of a particular skill.

- **Adults are self-directed learners.** Adults direct their own learning. They want to feel that they have some control over what they learn and the manner in which they learn it. Adults also need to feel that their opinions matter and their learning needs are respected.

- **Adults bring a variety of life experiences to any learning situation.** Such life experiences can facilitate any learning activity. Even experiences not directly related to healthcare can enhance education.

- **Adults concentrate on acquiring knowledge and skills that help them improve their professional and/or personal lives.** Adults measure the importance of education by focusing on how new knowledge and skills will help them improve their professional performance or enhance their private lives.

- **Adults respond to both extrinsic and intrinsic motivators.** Adults must know how learning activities meet their extrinsic and intrinsic needs. Extrinsic motivators include things such as job promotions and raises in salaries. Examples of intrinsic motivators include enhanced self-esteem and an increase in job satisfaction.

Learning styles

When you assess competency, you are often in the position of teacher. Even though a staff member demonstrates competency, you may have suggestions to help improve some aspect of his or her skill. Include an overview of learning styles when you design your competency assessment training program (Avillion 2004):

- **Auditory learners:** Auditory learners assimilate knowledge by hearing. They prefer lectures, discussions, and audiotapes. They respond most favorably to verbal instructions.

- **Visual learners:** Visual learning is the most predominant adult learning style. Visual learners sit in the front of a classroom, take detailed notes, and respond to verbal discussions that contain large amounts of imagery.

- **Kinesthetic learners:** Kinesthetic learners learn best by "doing." They need direct hands-on involvement and physical activity as part of the learning experience.

Maintaining objectivity

It is important that those who assess competency maintain their objectivity. The training program should contain information about performing objective evaluations and not letting personal feelings—positive or negative—influence the outcome of the assessment.

Offering constructive criticism

This is one of the most challenging responsibilities of anyone who evaluates the job performance of others. The purpose of constructive criticism is to provide feedback on both strengths and weaknesses. Constructive criticism should motivate, reinforce learning, and identify the nature and extent of problems. One of the most important parts of constructive criticism is the development of a specific plan to help staff members improve their performance. Use the following four steps when giving feedback:

1. **Identify the unacceptable actions.** What is the staff member doing or failing to do that is not acceptable? Remember to focus on the employee's behavior, *not* on his or her personality. Give specific examples, such as "You did not follow sterile techniques when you touched the IV tubing with your sterile-gloved hand," not "It seems as though you do not care whether you endanger the patient by ignoring proper sterile techniques."

2. **Explain the outcome.** What about the behavior is unacceptable? How does it negatively impact productivity, patient outcomes, and so on? Be specific. Use descriptive terms instead of evaluative terms.

3. **Establish the expectation.** What must the employee do to correct unacceptable behavior? Again, be specific, and use objective, descriptive terms. You are describing actions to improve behavior, not providing evaluative comments about a person's personality.

4. **Identify the consequences.** What will happen if the employee corrects his or her behavior? What will happen if he or she does not?

How to assess competency consistently

One of the biggest challenges of any competency assessment program is the need for consistency among those conducting the assessments. How do you make sure that one person is not too stringent and another too lenient? Are friends assessing friends' competency? Does this make a difference in the outcome? Are people who dislike each other assessing each other's competency? Your training program must provide staff members with the tools and support needed to conduct competency assessments properly. This includes maintaining up-to-date policies and procedures, appropriate documentation checklists, and adequate education and training (a detailed description of these components appears later in this chapter).

Consistency in documentation is as important as consistency in approach. Everyone should use the same tool template. A procedure that describes how to document competency is needed.

Identifying your competency assessors

Can you identify competency assessors by title? Let's look at some common job titles that may carry with them the responsibility for competency assessment.

- **Preceptors:** The ability to perform competency assessment is an integral part of the preceptor role. The preceptor is necessary to the successful orientation of new employees. The essential qualities needed by competency assessors are also preceptor attributes. These qualities include the following:
  – Possesses excellent clinical skills or, in nonclinical roles, excellence in job-specific skills
  – Demonstrates respect for colleagues
  – Acts as an excellent role model
  – Demonstrates outstanding interpersonal communication skills

  The assumption that preceptors adequately assess competency is based on the belief that your preceptor training program includes the essential components described earlier in this chapter. To increase the efficiency of training delivery, consider inviting staff members who need to be trained as competency assessors (but who are not preceptors) to the preceptor classes that offer training in competency assessment.

Chapter 4

- **Nurse managers:** Nurse managers are generally not the best people to assess clinical competency. In today's healthcare environment, nurse managers spend the majority of their time performing administrative duties such as staffing, budgeting, developing leadership, and handling performance issues. Their expertise in these areas, however, makes them able to validate such competencies in fellow nurse managers. Nurse managers rely on their staff members to possess clinical expertise, just as staff members rely on nurse managers for administrative expertise. Remember that to assess clinical competency properly, the evaluator must be able to demonstrate excellence in clinical skills. Nurse managers assess the managerial competency of their peers.

- **Staff development specialists:** Staff development specialists are the education experts within a healthcare organization. Their specific roles and areas of expertise determine whether they are involved in clinical competency assessment. For example, a staff development specialist based on the coronary-care unit who provides direct patient care as well as staff education is qualified to assess clinical competency. However, the staff development specialist who primarily offers management and leadership training and does not provide direct patient care is generally not qualified to assess clinical competency.

  Don't forget that staff development specialists must demonstrate competency in the adult education arena as well. Such competencies as program planning, teaching, and evaluating the effectiveness of education are essential to those who specialize in staff development.

  Staff development specialists work with management and the staff to design the organization's entire competency assessment program in addition to the program's training component. They provide the educational expertise that makes for a sound foundation for any competency program. But like anyone else who is responsible for assessing competency, staff development specialists must be competent in the skills that they evaluate.

- **Staff nurses:** Staff nurses who demonstrate the necessary skills may also be part of a competency assessment program. It is important that they receive the necessary training. Depending on the arrangement of your clinical ladder or other similar programs, you may choose to have competency assessment as part of the requirements for promotion.

- **Nursing assistants (NAs):** Can you think of exceptionally competent NAs in your organization? Training such NAs to assess the competency of their peers is a definite possibility. As you develop a promotional ladder for NAs, consider training those who are exceptional to participate in competency assessment.

- **Nonclinical staff:** Most healthcare organizations have competency assessment programs in place for nonclinical areas as well as for clinical areas. As your competency program develops and expands, don't forget to be on the lookout for nonclinical staff members who have what it takes to assess the competency of others.

You already know that you need to document competency achievement. Don't forget to document that your trainees have achieved competency in their ability to evaluate the performance of others. Figure 4.1 shows an example of a form that you can use for such documentation.

Chapter 4

Figure 4.1

Successful completion of competency assessment training form

Date: _____
Objectives: _____
_____
_____

Competency demonstration:
    1. Explains purpose and importance of a competency assessment program
    2. Incorporates the principles of adult learning as part of assessing competency
    3. Recognizes various learning styles and meets the needs of learners representing these styles
    4. Maintains objectivity when assessing competency
    5. Offers feedback in a constructive manner
    6. Is consistent in competency assessment approach
    7. Documents results of competency assessment accurately and consistently

Trainer comments:
_____
_____
_____

Learner comments:
_____
_____
_____

Competency assessment training was successfully completed:

_____   _____
Trainer's signature and date   Learner's signature and date

Competency assessment training was not successfully completed:

_____
Trainer's signature and date

The following steps will be taken by the learner to successfully complete training:

    Action   To be completed by the following date:
_____
_____
_____

_____
Learner's signature and date

Peer review

The word *peer* is defined as a person or thing having the same rank, value, and/or ability—in other words, an equal. If an important part of your competency program is the concept of "peer review," be careful that you are truly asking peers to evaluate peers. For example, suppose City Hospital's competency policy/procedure states that competency is assessed via a peer-review competency assessment program. City Hospital also has a career ladder for nurses that includes the following titles: staff nurse I, staff nurse II, and staff nurse III.

During a recent competency evaluation session, a staff nurse III (Carolyn) observes a staff nurse II (Amanda) performing the insertion of an intravenous needle. Carolyn documents that Amanda is not competent and needs remedial work. Amanda files a grievance with the hospital disciplinary board stating that Carolyn evaluated her unfairly. In part, the grievance reads, "As a staff nurse III, Carolyn held Amanda to a higher standard, instead of evaluating her according to her experience at the staff nurse II level. Because City Hospital maintains that competency assessment is a form of peer review, Amanda was unfairly evaluated." The disciplinary board supports Amanda, and Carolyn's competency assessment documentation is removed from Amanda's file.

Sound far-fetched? Unfortunately, this kind of problem is not uncommon. Let's look at some pitfalls that might have contributed to City Hospital's (and Carolyn's) dilemma. Consider the following questions/comments:

- Did the policy/procedure clearly define the concept of peer review? Could this problem have been avoided by stating that competency is assessed by several types of staff members (i.e., peers and those functioning at a higher level according to the organization's career ladder)? If the policy is written in this manner, Carolyn could assess the competency of peers, subordinates, and those at a lower level than she on the clinical ladder as long as she is competent in the skill being assessed.

- Did Carolyn receive appropriate training in how to assess competency? Are the results of this training documented?

- Was it clear what had to be accomplished for competency to be achieved? Were the steps in writing and were they part of the competency assessment documentation tool? Did both nurses clearly understand what had to be demonstrated?

Chapter 4

- Was objectivity maintained? Do interpersonal conflicts exist between Carolyn and Amanda?

Peer review is an excellent means of support and a worthwhile component of competency assessment. But be very careful that you define what you mean by a peer review. As in the case of City Hospital, if you fail to allow a more experienced nurse to evaluate a less experienced nurse or a subordinate, you may encounter serious problems. You may want to incorporate the definitions of various levels of expertise within your policies and procedures. Use the criteria established by your clinical ladder programs to delineate what levels of the staff are able to evaluate other levels of the staff. It may sound like a lot of extra work or that you're being overcautious, but this type of anticipatory planning prevents or reduces the number of grievances or union actions you encounter.

Keeping your validation system consistent

Nothing is as demoralizing as inconsistency in evaluation, and few things are as challenging as ensuring consistency of approach among many different people. Here are some tips for helping to maintain inter-rater reliability among your competency assessors:

- Select your competency assessor based on the characteristics described earlier in this chapter. You may be tempted to have all members of the nursing staff assess the competency of others. In this day and age of nursing shortages and the need for complex nursing interventions, having everyone assess competency may seem like a quick fix to the problem of documenting competency assessment, but don't succumb to this temptation. In the long run, it will lead to disgruntled employees, failure to adequately assess competency, and a plethora of union and disciplinary grievances. Establish your criteria for selection, put it in writing in policies and procedures, and stick to it.

- The ability to assess the competency of fellow employees is in itself a competency. Successful completion of the training program on competency assessment must be documented. Failure to successfully complete the program demands that the trainee perform remedial work. He or she must not assess the competency of others until training is successfully completed.

- Avoid compromising objectivity whenever possible. If competency is assessed individually in an on-the-job environment, avoid pairing staff members who have known interpersonal conflicts. Likewise, avoid pairing staff members who are close friends. Either situation runs the risk of accusations of favoritism or prejudice. Consider having staff members from other units evaluate each other. Doing so may enhance objectivity.

- Ensure that the steps that must be performed, along with descriptions regarding how they are to be performed, are clearly documented on the competency assessment form. Never assume that "everyone knows how to do this"! Failure to achieve competency can have dramatic consequences, including termination of employment. The only way to ensure consistency fairly is to provide a written guide delineating what constitutes successful competency demonstration.

- Develop a written checklist so that competency is evaluated on a step-by-step basis. The competency assessor must sign and date the checklist. The learner must also sign and date the checklist. Any remedial action plans must be documented along with targeted dates for achievement.

- The person assessing competency must document his or her evaluation findings. This task cannot be delegated to someone else. For example, suppose a busy manager asks one of her senior staff nurses to document a competency assessment for her. This is completely unacceptable. Competency assessment is just like any other type of nursing documentation: You do it, you document it.

- Have a plan in place to deal with persons who object to their competency rating. Include this plan in your policies and procedures. If a staff member is unfairly evaluated, he or she needs to know that there is a professional way to seek a reassessment. The steps that must be taken, including any necessary objective evidence, should be described in these policies and procedures.

- Policies and procedures must also describe the circumstances under which a grievance or other protest mechanism will be heard.

Chapter 4

Incorporating population-specific competencies

The Joint Commission changed its focus from age-specific to population-specific care. However, it does not define this term, but leaves it up to the individual institution to do so.

> **According to Webster's (Agnes 2006), the term *population-specific competency* might be defined as follows:**
>
> **Population** – a. all the people in a country, region, etc. b. a specified part of the people in a given area. c. the total set of persons.
>
> **Specific** – a. limiting or limited; precise. b. a characteristic of something. c. a special or particular kind.
>
> **Competency** – a. condition or quality of being competent. b. sufficient for one's needs.

The various physiological and psychological needs of each patient population group is part of any well-designed competency program. The ability to implement population-appropriate interventions is critical to the quality and suitability of patient care.

Most organizations serve a variety of populations and age ranges that can and often do require complex coordination and integration of care. Patient care is managed by staff members who are competent to address the needs of the patient population they serve; whether through case management which targets high-risk populations because of their various combinations of health, social, and functional problems, or through disease management which targets populations that generally have one major diagnosis and a relatively standard set of needs.

Many patient care units are designed based on specialty or specific patient populations. Patients are admitted to units where staff members are familiar with and competent to care for a select patient population as a result of their general, divisional, and unit/population-specific orientations and ongoing education/training and competency assessment. For example, patients requiring total hip replacement will most likely be admitted to an orthopedic unit, those with psychiatric disorders to a behavioral health unit, multiple-trauma patients to an ICU, high-risk pregnancy patients to the perinatal unit, and the list goes on. However, sometimes the complexity of a patient's care requires the skill and competence of a staff trained in several different specialties, necessitating collaboration among various interdisciplinary team members. Figure 4.2 includes examples of population-specific care.

Chapter 4

> **Figure 4.2**
>
> # Case Studies
>
> A 20-year-old 7-month pregnant woman was admitted to the Perinatal Unit with preeclampsia. Staff members working in this area have been specifically educated and skilled to care for pregnant women with this condition. Unfortunately, the patient did not respond to treatment, convulsed and underwent an emergency cesarean section for the delivery of a healthy baby girl. Clinical and laboratory studies revealed the onset of HELLP syndrome. Within a short period of time the patient became very unstable, requiring a transfer to the ICU. The ICU is staffed by those who have specialized education and skills to meet the needs of this now critically ill adult who required mechanical ventilation and placement of various monitoring devices that can only be used in critical care. For the next 10 days the ICU staff provided the bulk of this patient's care with frequent consultation and input into the plan of care provided by the Mother-Baby staff. Meanwhile the Special Care Nursery staff cared for the infant girl. On day 8, the patient showed much improvement and was transferred to the Mother-Baby unit and finally discharged to home.
>
> ---
>
> A 45-year-old woman with a history of psychiatric problems is admitted for management of a schizophrenic episode. While obtaining her health history, it is discovered that this patient underwent a gastric bypass procedure 6 months ago. She is unable to give a description of the surgical procedure or her current diet to the nurse admitting her. The nurse makes the admitting psychiatrist aware of the recent weight loss surgery procedure. The psychiatrist orders a consult from a Bariatric Surgeon and from the Bariatric Dietitian. The unit secretary calls the Bariatric Care Center to initiate the consult to the surgeon and to the dietitian. The Bariatric Surgeon completes the consult, and talks with the psychiatrist about the impact of the gastric bypass surgery on absorption of medications in the small intestine. The dietitian also sees the patient, and she contacts the dietary staff to make them aware that this patient requires a specific gastric bypass diet. She provides education to the staff regarding the surgery and the reason that this diet is needed, and she makes sure that the orders are entered correctly. She also makes certain that the patient's nurse understands how to verify that the tray is correct when it arrives on the floor. A copy of the consult is provided by the surgeon to the Bariatric Case Manager for the patient's outpatient chart, and the dietitian writes a note in the inpatient chart and the outpatient chart each time she sees the patient. The surgeon requests that the patient be seen in the Bariatric Care Center for follow-up within two weeks of discharge from the hospital.
>
> ---
>
> A 19-year-old male arrives at Same Day Surgery according to standard protocol to undergo gastric bypass surgery. He is extremely obese, with a weight of almost 500 pounds, and arrangements were made in advance for a Hillrom Total Care bed. Upon arrival in the OR, the surgical coordinator observes that the Total Care bed is not available. Knowing that all bariatric patients who exceed 350 pounds must be placed on the Total Care bed, she contacts Distribution to have the bed delivered right away. The

> **Figure 4.2**
>
> ## Case Studies (cont.)
>
> staff in Distribution, who are also aware of the policy for use of the Total Care bed with bariatric surgery patients, make sure that the bed is taken to the OR within 30 minutes so that it is ready for the patient upon completion of surgery. The patient is moved to the bed while still in the OR, and is ultimately transferred to the inpatient unit on the correct bed. The following morning, again according to protocol, an Upper GI study is ordered for 7:30 am. Upon arrival on the floor, the transporter realizes that the wheelchair he brought is the standard size, and will not accommodate this patient. He thoughtfully does not make note of this in front of the patient, but knowing that there must not be a delay in getting this patient to radiology, goes to the desk and calls down to his department to have a bariatric wheelchair brought up immediately. Another member of the Transportation Department arrives in 15 minutes with a wheelchair, which is appropriate for transportation of a patient of this size, and the patient is safely delivered to Radiology on time for his procedure.
>
> *Source: Summa Health System Hospital, Akron, OH. Reprinted with permission.*

Chapter 4

The demonstration and corresponding documentation of population-specific staff competencies are important for a number of reasons. First, such competency validates the knowledge and skills of staff members. Appropriate knowledge and skills contribute to the quality of patient care and family services. And finally, The Joint Commission requires that population-specific competency be assessed on an ongoing basis and that the findings of these assessments are documented and maintained as part of the employee's file.

Population-specific competency requires proof of education and training, as well as the demonstration of skill achievement. During orientation, all employees must receive education and training concerning the specific patient age groups for which they will provide care. Remember that this includes employees who, although not new to your organization, are new to a department or unit. For example, suppose that Martha has worked on an adult oncology unit for five years. She is transferring to a pediatric oncology unit this month. During Martha's orientation to pediatric oncology, the organization must provide her with education and training specific to pediatric oncology patients. This education and training must be documented and maintained in Martha's employee file.

Does population-specific competency mean that all caregivers must demonstrate competency of all types of patients? No, this is not the case. Identify the age range of patients that staff members encounter most frequently in their work.

For example, a nurse who works on an adult oncology unit cares for patients in the young adult through geriatric age ranges. She or he must demonstrate competency in providing nursing care to patients who are young adults, middle-aged adults, and geriatric adults. Likewise, a nurse who works in a neonatal ICU would need to demonstrate competency in providing care for neonates, not geriatric patients.

What are some efficient, cost-effective ways to achieve and demonstrate population-specific competencies? Let's start with education and training.

Simply attending an education program does not guarantee transfer of learning to the work setting. However, because healthcare science and research seems to bring new and exciting discoveries to the healthcare arena every day, part of the requirement of competency maintenance may involve participating in a specified number of age-specific education hours. These hours do not need to be offered exclusively in a classroom setting. Options such as self-learning packets, videos, and computer-based learning are cost-effective, efficient ways to deliver education and training. Successful achievement of educational posttests measures learning or the acquisition of knowledge.

But as we discussed earlier in this chapter, knowledge acquisition does not equate to the ability to successfully transfer knowledge. How can we assess population-specific competencies? Ongoing competency may be evaluated in several ways, including direct observation, medical record review, and patient outcomes. Let's review the competency of Melanie, a nurse who works on an adult medical-surgical unit. What methodologies can we use to be sure that she is competent in providing care to geriatric patients?

- **Medical record review:** Are appropriate skin care nursing interventions documented? Is there documented evidence that safety measures are in place considering the patient's diagnosis? Has skin turgor been assessed? Identify specific interventions for the assessor to find within the medical record, including nursing care plans, nurses' notes, and so on. You need to be specific to facilitate consistency of evaluation.

- **Direct observations:** Does Melanie provide care in a manner that incorporates age-specific concerns for the geriatric patient? In addition to observing Melanie as she actually provides care, you can assess patient outcomes and the environment. For instance, when assessing safety issues, determine whether the call bell is within reach, whether nonskid slippers are readily available, and so on. Again, be specific about what assessors need to evaluate. Select some universal geriatric issues and determine whether these issues are part of the patient's plan of care.

- **Equipment use:** Is equipment use adapted to the needs of the geriatric patient? For instance, if a geriatric patient is receiving intravenous hydration, are measures taken to avoid fluid overload, a potential danger for an elderly patient?

These are only a few of the ways to assess age-related competency. Remember that all reviewers must carry out such assessments in a consistent manner. This means that written guidelines must be established.

Chapter 4

Documentation and recordkeeping

It is essential that your competency assessment program include appropriate documentation and maintenance of such documentation. Various sample checklists and templates are presented throughout this chapter. As a summary of important issues, let's review documentation components that are absolutely essential:

- **Assessment documentation must be dated.** Although you may think that this component is self-evident, it is astonishing how many times it is missed. The top of any form generally contains a space for the date, but all signatures should be dated as well. This decreases the chance of any discrepancies concerning assessment dates.

- **Identify the specific competency being assessed.** This includes the specific age ranges assessed as part of age-specific competencies.

- **Identify the objectives that must be achieved to demonstrate competency.** These objectives should be written in measurable terms and contain action verbs such as *performs, identifies, demonstrates*, and so forth. Nonmeasurable terms such as *understand, be aware of,* and so forth are to be avoided.

- **Document specific steps in competency achievement.** Consistency cannot be ensured unless the specific, step-by-step actions that must be performed to achieve competency are in writing. All assessors must have the same expectations of the people they are evaluating.

- **Document the methods used to assess competency.** Possible methods include observation of direct patient care, medical record review, and evaluation of the patient's environment. Again, don't forget to identify what the assessor must look for in the selected method(s).

- **Document remedial action.** If competency is not achieved, document the remedial actions that will be taken to help the learner achieve competency. The actions should be specific and should include target achievement dates.

Conclusion

Competency assessment is an integral part of your patient-care delivery system. Those who assess the competency of others must receive appropriate education and training so that they are effective, efficient, and consistent in their approach.

Careful, objective documentation of such education and training is as important as documentation of competency assessment itself. In fact, achievement as a competency assessor is a competency too. Select with care those individuals who assess competency. Not every staff member is suited to assess and facilitate learning in others. Clinical excellence does not equate to the ability to facilitate the job performance of colleagues.

The templates and forms presented in this chapter are intended to be starting points for the customization of your own tools. Adapt them to meet the needs of your staff members.

Finally, remember that competency assessment is a learning tool as well as a means of validation. Use these opportunities to facilitate the continuing education and professional development of staff members, with the ultimate goal being improved patient outcomes.

REFERENCES

1. Agnes, Michael. (Ed). (2006). *Webster's New World College Dictionary*. Cleveland: Wiley Publishing.

2. Avillion, Adrianne E. (2004). *A Practical Guide to Staff Development: Tools and Techniques for Effective Education*. Marblehead, MA: HCPro, Inc.

3. Avillion, Adrianne E., Barbara Brunt, and Mary Jane Ferrell. (2007). *Nursing Professional Development Review and Resource Manual*. Silver Spring, MD: Institute for Credentialing Innovation.

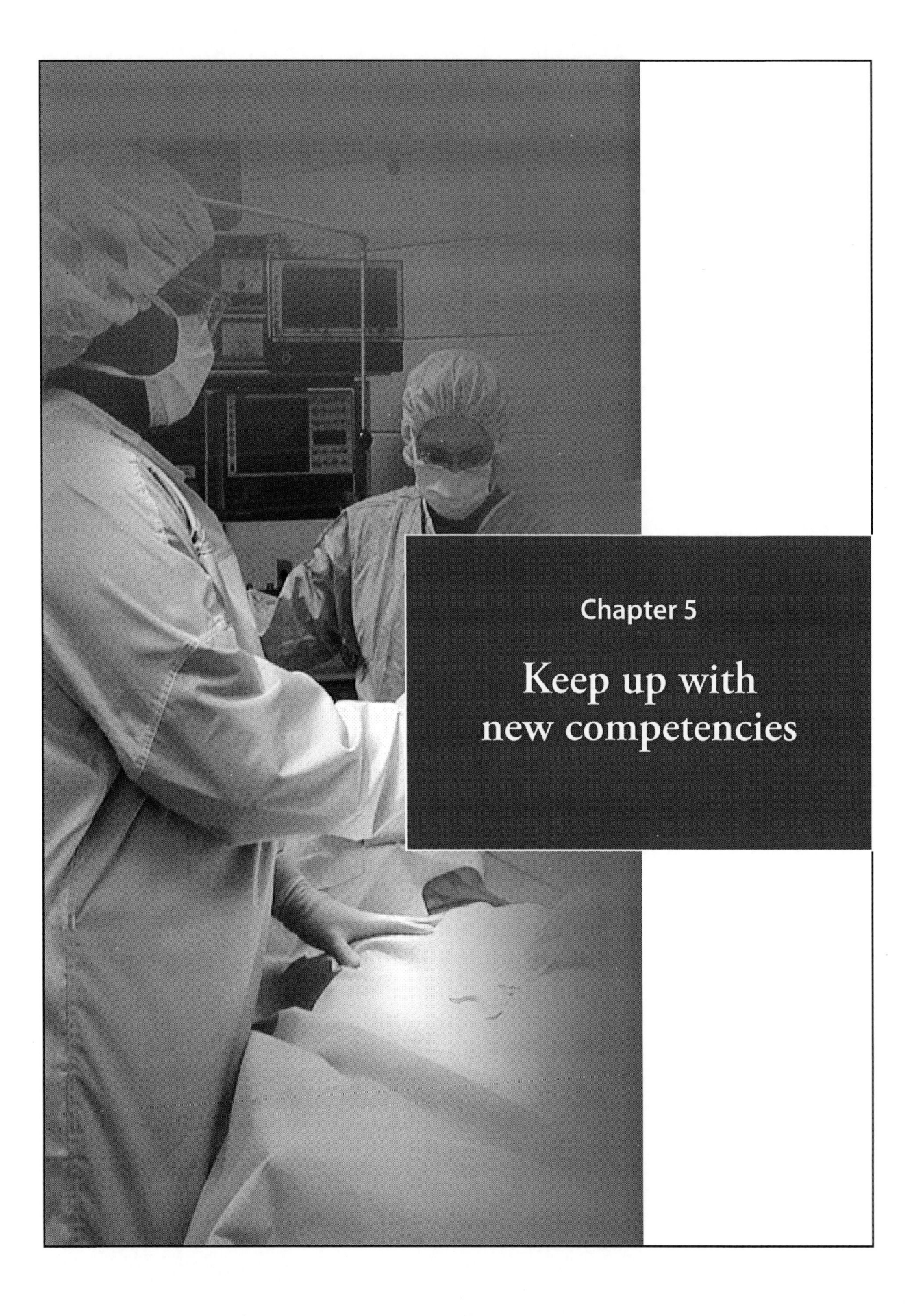

Chapter 5

Keep up with new competencies

Chapter 5

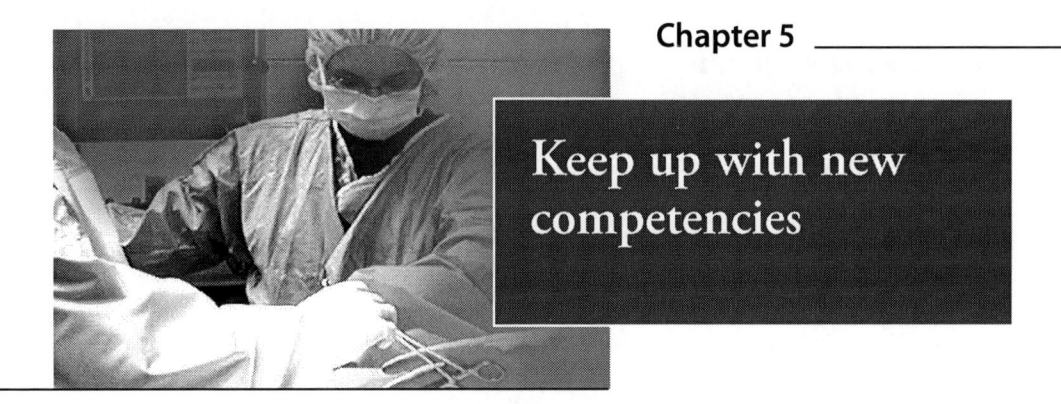

Keep up with new competencies

Learning objectives

After reading this chapter, the participant should be able to:

- List potential categories for new competencies
- Identify best practices for implementing new competencies
- Discuss dimensions of competencies

Hundreds of new concerns arise in healthcare daily. How do you determine which ones become competencies?

Let's start by describing what a competency is not. Competencies are not required for every new piece of equipment, every new or revised policy and procedure, every interpersonal communication problem, or every skill that accompanies a specific job description. However, a competency is a skill that significantly affects or has the potential to significantly affect the patient. Such issues may fall under the categories of psychomotor skills or interpersonal skills.

Doesn't everything in healthcare have the potential to significantly affect a patient? Technically, yes. But if you define the word *significant* that broadly, you will have so many competencies that you'll drown in paperwork, and it will become impossible to assess that many items efficiently.

Potential categories for new competencies

Let's look at some general categories that have the potential for competency development.

New equipment

Not every piece of new equipment triggers the need for a competency. In most cases, a simple inservice suffices. For example, suppose your organization orders new patient beds. The beds have some additional features that the old beds lacked, and an inservice is conducted to orient staff members to work safely with these new beds. Now suppose that new equipment including Circoelectric beds, Bradford frames, and Stryker frames arrives for your organization's newly opened rehabilitation unit. These devices require special skills to ensure patient safety and will be used often, although not daily. These types of new equipment are more suitable for ongoing competency development. They have significant patient impact, require a high level of skill and safety awareness, and are in frequent use.

When new equipment arrives, ask yourself these questions:

- Does the equipment require high levels of skill to operate?

- Who will operate the new equipment? Must the staff have special qualifications (e.g., RN designation) to use this equipment?

- What potential patient safety risks are associated with the new equipment?

- How often will the new equipment be in use?

If you find that equipment requires qualified staff members to have high levels of skill, is associated with significant patient safety issues, and is used often enough that the staff is able to maintain competency, the equipment may require the development of a competency.

Interpersonal communications

Interpersonal communications are the foundation of healthcare interventions. From the first contact at a reception desk or admission's office through and including communication with physicians, nurses, and therapists, interpersonal interaction influences the patient's healthcare experience.

How would you rate interpersonal communication skills among your colleagues? Does risk management/ quality improvement data indicate any negative trends in this arena? Do staff members encounter hostility from patients/families? This is not uncommon, especially in areas such as the emergency department, head trauma unit, and inpatient mental health unit. But how do you assess this type of competency? It is not a step-by-step psychomotor skill. However, there are options.

Direct observation is one such option. Keep in mind, however, that written guidelines are necessary for the person assessing competency. Additional observations may be set up in a "competency skills lab" where staff members must respond to various types of behavior in role-play situations. These are not conducted in the actual work setting, but they may be a useful addendum to direct observation.

Be creative when assessing nontechnical skills such as these. Another validation option is to conduct mock drills involving staff members playing the role of agitated/violent patients or family members. These have the advantage of surprise and may be more valuable than a controlled role-play situation.

New patient populations

The appearance of new diseases and syndromes requires the implementation of new diagnostic and treatment interventions. The AIDS epidemic changed almost every aspect of healthcare and triggered the need for universal precautions and more secure protective equipment. The development of new drugs to combat this syndrome requires that healthcare professionals add to the ever-growing body of knowledge concerning medications, their actions, and potential side effects. Similarly, until recently, few healthcare professionals had ever heard of severe acute respiratory syndrome (also known as SARS). Now it is a household term.

The point is that new patient populations require new knowledge and the application of that knowledge in the healthcare setting. As you evaluate the need for new skills to apply this knowledge, you are also evaluating the need for additional competency development. However, stick to the recommendations made earlier in this chapter. Consider the level of knowledge and skill needed, how often the knowledge will be applied, and the effect of these newly acquired skills on patient outcomes.

New treatment measures

Thanks to intense research and scientific inquiry, we are able to treat and even cure illnesses and catastrophic injuries that were untreatable just a few short years ago. With these healthcare advances come new bodies of knowledge and the need to use that knowledge safely and efficiently. As new treatment measures become necessary to your organization's ability to provide patient services, so does the need for additional competency development.

Remember that you don't need to keep the same competencies forever. Perhaps new treatments and equipment and the demise or reduction of certain illnesses (e.g., polio) trigger the need for you to delete certain competencies from your program. As you evaluate the need for new competencies, don't forget to evaluate the need to streamline those already in existence.

New medications

The U.S. Food and Drug Administration approves significant numbers of new medications annually. Most of them do not require competency development; however, some drugs require special knowledge, and administration techniques for these drugs necessitate competency development. Use your guidelines of skill level, patient impact, and frequency of use to determine the need for new competencies.

Research endeavors

If your organization is a research site, your staff members may be exposed to new (and sometimes dangerous) ways of treating illnesses and injuries more often than the average healthcare worker. Examine your research policies and procedures. Which staff members frequently initiate experimental treatments, including medication administration? How do you measure their competency to initiate these treatments? As you evaluate your competency assessment program, don't forget to pay close attention to the research conducted at your organization: The resultant treatment initiatives could mandate the development of new competencies.

Guidelines for new competency development

Develop a policy that guides your competency assessment program (Avillion 2004). Part of that policy describes your guidelines for new competency development (and for the deletion of competencies that are no longer necessary).

Answer the following questions to identify what to incorporate into your organization's policy:

- What new diagnostic tests, treatments, or other factors are developed that require staff members to add to their knowledge and expertise?

- What current competencies no longer meet the criteria for ongoing competency assessment? Are the treatments outdated, are they no longer initiated, or have they become part of a daily routine with reduced impact on patient outcome and little or no exceptional level of skill?

- What level of skill do new initiatives require?

- Who is authorized to perform/evaluate the effectiveness of new initiatives?

- What safety risks (to patients, visitors, and staff members) are associated with these new initiatives?

- How often will these new initiatives be implemented?

Think about your answer to the last question carefully. Staff members cannot achieve or retain competency unless they have fairly regular opportunities to use new knowledge and skills. Consider the following example:

A newly opened, freestanding 100-bed rehabilitation facility does not have 24-hour physician coverage on-site. The patient population consists primarily of spinal cord injury, stroke, traumatic head injury, hip fracture, multiple fracture, and amputee patients. Although the patients are relatively stable prior to their transfer to the facility, occasionally a patient deteriorates rapidly and emergency medical services (EMS) is notified. Patients also go into cardiac arrest. All direct patient care providers are CPR-certified. In the event of cardiac arrest, CPR is initiated and an IV is started, and the use of a portable defibrillator is sanctioned if warranted. This procedure was developed with the assistance of EMS personnel. The arrival of the EMS squad from the local acute-care health system takes between seven and 10 minutes.

The administrative staff (CEO, director of nursing, and comptroller) expressed concern that patients could not be intubated and advance life support drugs administered prior to the arrival of the EMS squad. They decided to mandate that all RNs working at the rehabilitation facility achieve and maintain advanced cardiac life support (ACLS) certification. These nurses, on the rare occasion of a cardiac arrest, would be expected to intubate patients and initiate ACLS treatment measures, including the administration of cardiac medications. The RNs would need to demonstrate ongoing competency in ACLS to keep their jobs. Is this a realistic competency?

Chapter 5

The answer, of course, is no. Nurses cannot maintain competency in a procedure as complex as ACLS when they do not have regular opportunities to use such knowledge and skills. In fact, attempting to intubate a patient when you have an opportunity to do so only once a year is extremely dangerous.

The EMS representatives teamed up with the facility's staff development specialists to convince the administrative staff that attempting to mandate ACLS certification would do more harm than good. But until this was accomplished, the nursing staff was quite upset, and some even resigned rather than attempt to achieve ACLS certification.

This example illustrates the importance of being able to use knowledge and apply skills to achieve and maintain competency. Knowledge acquisition alone is not enough.

The checklist in Figure 5.1 may help you to document your assessment of the need for new competency development.

Figure 5.1

New competency assessment checklist

Date: _____

Item being evaluated:
- ❏ New equipment
- ❏ New treatment
- ❏ New medication
- ❏ New patient population
- ❏ Interpersonal communication issue
- ❏ Research initiatives

Identify the item specifically (e.g., type and purpose of equipment, description of new treatment, etc.).
_____
_____
_____

1. What new knowledge/skills are required to safely initiate this new item?
_____
_____
_____

2. Who is authorized to perform these new skills (e.g., RNs, LPNs, etc.)
_____
_____
_____

3. What, if any, quality improvement/risk management data indicate a need for this competency?
_____
_____
_____

4. What risks to patients, visitors, and staff members are associated with the new initiative?
_____
_____
_____

5. How often will staff members have an opportunity to apply the new knowledge and skills necessary for safe, accurate implementation of this new initiative?
_____
_____
_____

Chapter 5

> **Figure 5.1**
>
> ## New competency assessment checklist (cont.)
>
> **There is a need for new competency development. The new competency is:**
> _____
> _____
> _____
>
> _____
> **Signature, title, and date**
>
> **There is no need for new competency development. The rationale for this is:**
> _____
> _____
> _____
>
> _____
> **Signature, title, and date**

Best practices for the implementation of new competencies

Unfortunately, new competencies do not evolve neatly on an annual basis, allowing ample time for appropriate education and training to occur. They pop up at any time, with varying degrees of urgency. Here are some suggestions for implementing new competencies (Cooper 2002).

Competency skills fairs

Some organizations have implemented day-long or half-day competency assessment days. These are called by various names, such as "skills fairs," "competency days," "competency skills labs," and so on. The premise is generally the same: A variety of competencies are assessed during a specified period and at an identified general location (usually a classroom setting). These events can be held at specified times throughout the year, such as annually, semiannually, or quarterly.

Advantages of this approach include the following:

- **Efficiency:** Competency days allow you to address the maximum number of people with a minimum number of observers.

- **Regular scheduling:** Staff members know when these events will occur and, in conjunction with their managers, can plan their attendance. Likewise, those responsible for organizing the competency days have planning time and the chance to add/delete competencies.

- **Decreased time away from the actual work site:** By planning regular assessment days, staffing needs can be planned in advance.

Disadvantages of this approach include the following:

- Competencies are added or deleted only at specific times throughout the year. This may compromise the timeliness of critical competency assessments.

- Competencies that require demonstration of actual patient-care interactions/procedures are not suitable for this approach.

- Having sufficient competency assessors on hand can be problematic.

- The length of time the fair is open can be a challenge. Twenty-four-hour availability requires a large number of competency assessors. If 24-hour availability is not possible, determining the hours

Chapter 5

of operation can draw complaints from staff members who must attend on their off time. In addition, because competency assessment is a mandate, staff members are entitled to be paid for attending these types of events, which can place a considerable burden on the organization's budget.

Drills and simulations

An evaluation form must be completed after each drill. This form serves as a record of behavior, a competency assessment, and a format to document strengths and areas for improvement. Examples of drills and simulations include mock codes, internal and external disasters, and hazardous-spill cleanup.

Drills and simulations:

- Require little or no additional staffing
- Can serve as a complement to the annual review of the environment of care plans required by the Occupational Safety & Health Administration
- Evaluate behavior in true-to-life situations

Disadvantages of drills and simulations are that they:

- May disrupt other programs or patient-care activities
- Require exceptionally well-qualified evaluators
- Need specific identification of required behaviors on evaluation forms

Performance improvement monitors

This approach relies on data from performance improvement (PI) documentation. PI indicators are useful when evaluating both interpersonal competencies and abilities to perform clinical skills.

Advantages of using PI monitors include the following:

- PI monitors are regular, reliable sources of data
- No additional time burden is required to collect the data
- Managers can simultaneously validate competency and complete a mandated activity without additional work, making the process more efficient

Disadvantages of using PI monitors include the following:

- They require the assumption that the PI data is accurate and objective

- They do not guarantee that competency was consistently evaluated if multiple people had input into the performance evaluation

Return demonstration/observation

Return demonstration can take place during the previously mentioned skills fair or on the job, which involves direct observation of skill performance.

Return demonstration/observation:

- Allows the assessor to actually see behavior and the employee's application of knowledge

- Allows for demonstration of new knowledge and skills in the actual work environment in "real-life" settings

Disadvantages of return demonstration/observation include the following:

- It may influence the behavior of the staff member being assessed because he or she is aware that an evaluation is taking place

- It cannot guarantee that employees' behavior is the same during the return demonstration/observation as when not being observed

Self-assessment

Self-assessment generally requires that employees complete a written exercise designed to identify their beliefs and knowledge about their job performance. The employees' assessment is compared to the managers' and other assessors' assessments. Any disparity must be addressed so that job performance improves.

Self-assessment:

- Helps employees to recognize their own beliefs and values and how these issues may affect their job performance

- Identifies incongruence between employees' beliefs and values and the organization's mission, vision, and values

Disadvantages of self-assessment include the following:

- It does not provide an opportunity for evaluation of the actual behaviors
- Results are influenced by employees' and assessors' personal values and beliefs
- Failure to address incongruence results in employees continuing to behave in ways that are inconsistent with the organization's mission, vision, and values

Dimensions of competencies

Each approach is distinct and focuses on specific aspects of employee skills. According to *Competency Assessment: A Practical Guide to the JCAHO Standards, Second edition* (Summers et al 2004), competencies are designed to evaluate particular features of skills, called *dimensions*. Each dimension includes explicit skills and knowledge. They include the following:

- *Critical-thinking dimension: the ability to use information or knowledge, including:*
  - Problem-solving
  - Planning
  - Clinical reasoning
  - Adapting to/facilitating change
  - Time management
  - Fiscal responsibility

- *Interpersonal dimension: the ability to work effectively with others, including:*
  - Communication
  - Conflict management
  - Customer service
  - Working effectively with members of various cultures and racial and ethnic backgrounds
  - Working as effective team players

- *Technical dimension: the possession of knowledge and the ability to use that knowledge to perform fine and gross motor functions, including:*
  - Cognitive abilities
  - Acquired knowledge
  - Psychomotor ability
  - Technical competence

As you evaluate the need for new competencies, review these dimensions to determine both need and approach. Remember that a competency assessment program focuses on verifying and validating skills and knowledge application in the workplace. The purpose of a competency program is to:

- Improve job performance
- Enhance patient outcomes
- Promote economic efficiency
- Increase organizational effectiveness

Demonstrated achievement of these goals shows that your competency assessment program is one that not only validates knowledge and skills, but also results in improved patient outcomes.

REFERENCES

1. Avillion A. 2004. *A Practical Guide to Staff Development: Tools and Techniques for Effective Education*. Marblehead, MA: HCPro, Inc.

2. Cooper, D. 2002. "The 'C' Word: Competency" in Kristen L. O'Shea, *Staff Development Nursing Secrets*. Philadelphia: Hanley & Belfus.

3. Summers, B., Tracy, J., and Woods, W. 2004. *Competency Assessment: A Practical Guide to the JCAHO Standards, Second Edition*. Marblehead, MA: HCPro, Inc.

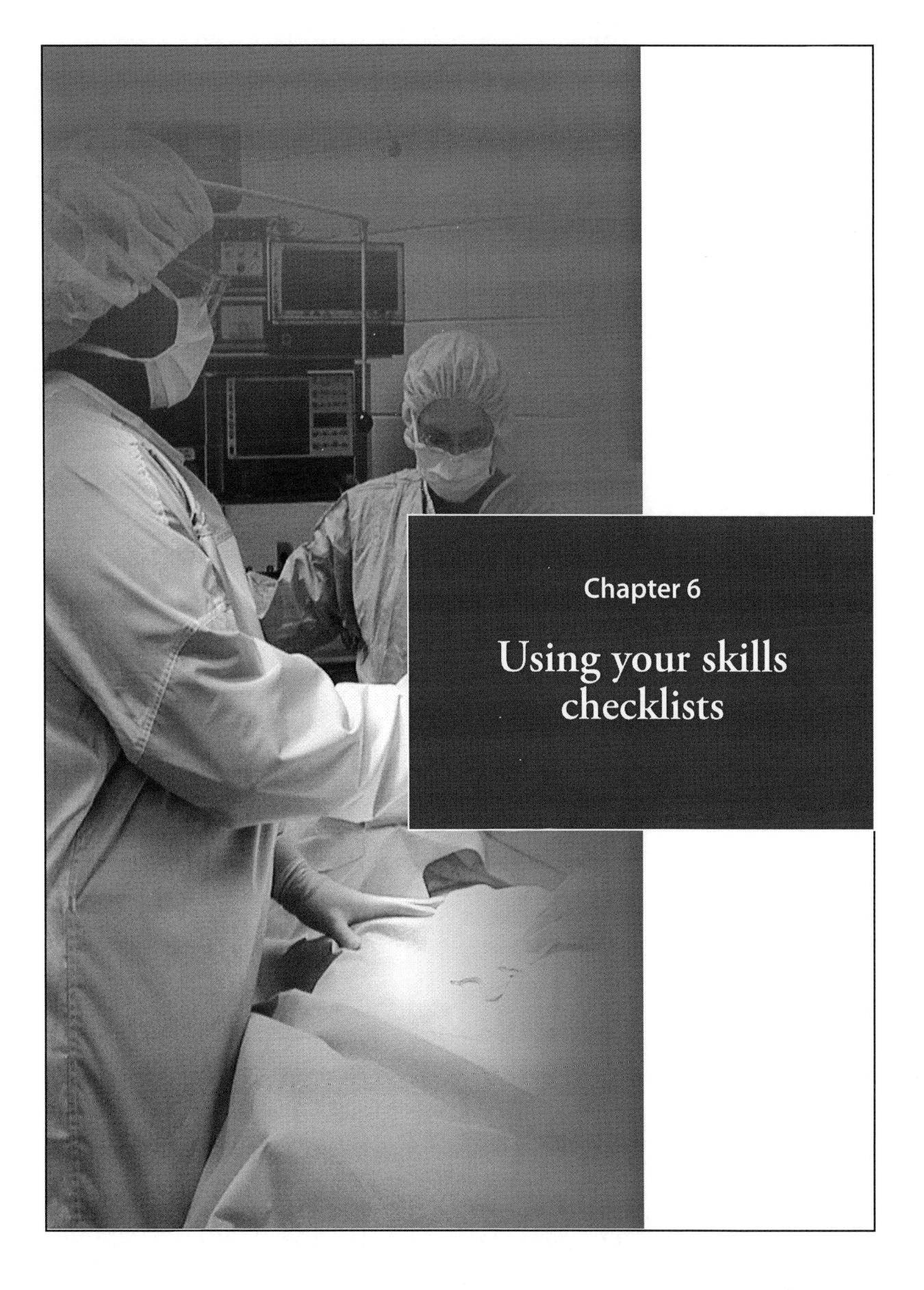

Chapter 6

Using your skills checklists

Chapter 6

Using your skills checklists

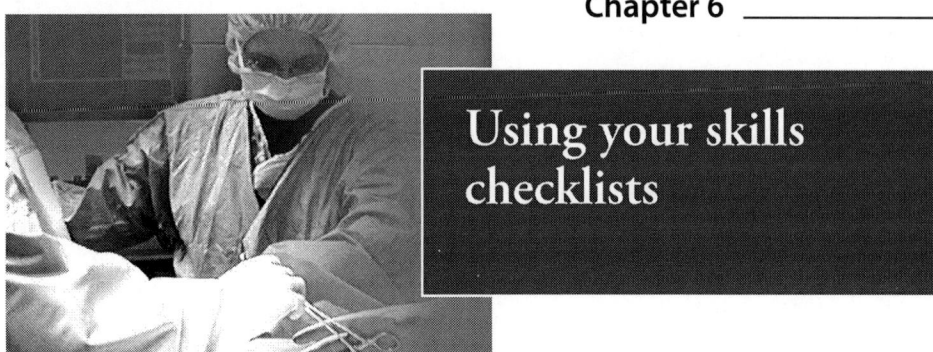

Learning objectives

After reading this chapter, the participant should be able to:

- Differentiate between difference between orientation checklists and skills checklists

Skills checklists must clearly identify expectations and should be completed by staff members who know how to use them. Criteria for safe, effective performance must be clearly defined, and everyone participating in the evaluation process must have a common understanding of the criteria and the basis for assigning ratings. Research has shown that if evaluators make direct observations using precise measurement criteria in checklists, with immediate feedback on performance, this is more effective than the traditional evaluation of clinical skills using subjective rating forms. The format for skills checklists may vary, but most contain similar information. Regardless of how they are used, skills checklists should:

- Be learner-oriented

- Focus on behaviors

- Be measurable

- Use criteria validated by experts

- Be specific enough to avoid ambiguity

Chapter 6

A template used to create the skills checklists included in this manual appears in Figure 6.1, and an electronic version of this template appears on your accompanying CD-ROM; you can open it as a Microsoft Word document. The individual's name and date are important to identify whose skills are being validated and when the evaluation is being conducted.

Using your skills checklists

Figure 6.1

Skills checklist template

Name: _____ Date: _____

Skill: [   ]

Steps	Completed	Comments

Self-assessment	Evaluation/ validation methods	Levels	Type of validation	Comments
❏ Experienced ❏ Need practice ❏ Never done ❏ Not applicable (based on scope of practice)	❏ Verbal ❏ Demonstration/ observation ❏ Practical exercise ❏ Interactive class	❏ Beginner ❏ Intermediate ❏ Expert	❏ Orientation ❏ Annual ❏ Other _____	

_____   _____
Employee signature   *Observer signature*

Evidence-Based Competency Management for the Medical-Surgical Unit, Second Edition

Chapter 6

The steps identified in the checklist should define the critical behaviors needed for effective performance of the skill and do not include every step of the procedure. You can use the "Completed" column to indicate that each step was performed correctly, but note that some checklists use a met/not met format instead. It is helpful if checklists include an area for comments. Also note that most checklists are used to evaluate a single occurrence.

In the checklist format just described, the self-assessment can give the evaluator an idea of the individual's perceived skill level, although that can never take the place of validating competency. Individuals may have different perceptions of their abilities that may or may not be consistent with the evaluator's perceptions. For instance, one person could indicate that he or she needs practice, even though that person is familiar and competent with that skill but is not familiar with the institution's policy and procedure. Another staff member could indicate that he or she needs practice because the staff member has performed the skill only once during his or her career. All required skills must be validated, regardless of the individual's assessment of his or her ability.

The evaluation/validation method areas indicate how the validation was performed. The method used most often is demonstration or observation of the individual performing the skill, but verbal questioning can also be effective in identifying the thought processes or critical thinking involved with skills. Practical exercises and interactive class activities can also be useful as validation methods.

The appropriate level (beginner, intermediate, or expert) can be indicated, as well as the type of validation. It is important to identify whether the assessment is part of an individual's orientation or whether it is an ongoing annual validation. It is also important that you have both the employee and the observer sign the checklist.

The Joint Commission mandates that all employees have their competence assessed upon hire and throughout their employment. One way to meet this standard is to have orientation checklists in addition to skills checklists (Joint Commission Resources 2008).

Differences between orientation checklists and skills checklists

Orientation checklists specify the knowledge, attitudes, and skills needed to perform safely. The information for an orientation checklist would come from the position description for that job classification and would outline the essential competencies for safe practice in that role. Skills checklists, on the other hand, include the specific tasks related to a policy or procedure. Skills checklists are often used to document ongoing competency, as compared to orientation checklists, which document initial competency.

Developing orientation checklists

Key elements in developing an orientation checklist are the job description and performance evaluation criteria. The components of the orientation program provide the framework. Essential information in the checklist would include the individual's name and the names of all evaluators. The hire date and unit are helpful to identify when the individual started in his or her role. Orientation checklists provide documentation of the initial assessment of competence required by The Joint Commission, as well as the individual's self-assessment. If evaluation during the orientation is a shared responsibility (e.g., with staff development educators and unit preceptors), different columns can be used to identify what was done during a classroom orientation and what was done in the clinical area. A "Not Evaluated" or "Not Applicable" column can be helpful for those skills that an orientee did not have an opportunity to perform during the orientation process.

Sample checklists for RN orientation (Figure 6.2) and nursing assistant (NA) orientation (Figure 6.3) are included as examples.

Orientation checklists should be developed with input from the management staff. This will ensure that they include the essential skills expected from the position. Generally, staff development personnel/preceptors complete orientation checklists. Preceptors help new employees adjust to the workplace and clinical unit, and they work with new employees to help plan the learning experiences and share knowledge of expected behaviors. They can help to reduce stress and enhance learning for new employees by using adult learning principles, documenting skill acquisition, and helping the new person socialize into the unit culture. The checklist helps to make employees accountable for their learning by clearly identifying expectations to be completed during the orientation period. After the orientation checklist is completed, it usually becomes part of the employee's permanent file, which protects both the employer and the employee.

Chapter 6

Figure 6.2

Competency-based orientation checklist

SUMMA HEALTH SYSTEM STAFF DEVELOPMENT
RN SKILLS ASSESSMENT/EVALUATION

NAME: _____ HIRE DATE: _____
UNIT: _____

STAFF DEVELOPMENT: INITIALS: PRECEPTORS: INITIALS:
_____   _____   _____   _____
_____   _____   _____   _____
_____   _____   _____   _____
_____   _____
_____   _____

Directions:

Orientee: Complete the self-assessment by placing a check (✓) in the appropriate column based on your level of familiarity or experience with each competency.

Staff Development/Preceptor: Complete the evaluation section for each competency after the orientee has demonstrated successful completion of that competency. Place the date and your initials in the appropriate column. If NE (not evaluated) is checked, include an explanation in the comments column.

	SELF-ASSESSMENT			EVALUATION			
Competencies	Comfortable	Need Review	Have never done	*SD ORT	Unit	**NE	Comments
I. Competency A. Applies a systematic problem-solving approach in the implementation of nursing plans of care:							
1. Uses nursing process to systematically assess, plan, implement and evaluate nursing care.							

*SD ORT = Staff Development Orientation **NE = If Not Evaluated, indicate explanation

Figure 6.2

Competency-based orientation checklist (cont.)

2. Provide/documents patient teaching/ discharge planning.							
3. Involves patient/ significant other in plan of care.							
4. Prioritizes nursing care for a group of patients.							
5. Initiates patient referrals as needed.							
6. Utilizes appropriate resources.							
B. Intravenous therapy 1. Initiates intravenous							
2. Monitors intravenous according to policy and procedure a. Checks rate							
b. Assesses for signs and symptoms of complications							
c. Initiates PRN adapter							
3. Uses infusion pumps correctly: • PCA							
• Baxter							
4. Draws blood specimens: • Routine							
• Central line							
• Blood cultures							
5. Administers blood and blood components.							

*SD ORT = Staff Development Orientation **NE = If Not Evaluated, indicate explanation

Chapter 6

Figure 6.2

Competency-based orientation checklist (cont.)

6. Maintains central line/ hyperalimentation.						
7. Applies/changes central line dressing.						
8. Administers IV medications (I.V.P.B. IV push).						
9. Documents administration of IV Therapy.						
10. Completes IV Therapy exam with a minimum score of 80%						
C. Medication administration 1. Describes usual dose, common side effects, compatibilities, action, and untoward reactions of medications.						
2. Administers medications						
a. I.M.						
b. SQ and Insulin						
c. Calculations						
d. Other						
3. Documents administration of medications (MAR, controlled drugs, etc.).						
4. Identifies medication error reporting system.						
D. Treatment and procedures 1. Inserts and maintains gastric feeding tubes.						

*SD ORT = Staff Development Orientation **NE = If Not Evaluated, indicate explanation

Figure 6.2

Competency-based orientation checklist (cont.)

2. Inserts and maintains urinary catheters.						
3. Performs trach care and suctioning.						
4. Assesses patient safety including proper utilization of restraints.						
5. Completes tissue therapy SLP.						
6. Provides and documents pre-and postop nursing care.						
7. Incorporates nursing measures to reduce and prevent the spread of infection in daily nursing care.						
8. Completes American Heart Association guidelines for BLS-C in CPR.						
9. Changes oxygen gauge and sets rate.						
10. Locates various items on the emergency cart.						
11. Identifies nursing responsibilities in emergency situations.						
12. Completes: a. Admission of patient						
b. Transfer of a patient						
c. Discharge of a patient						
13. Performs neurological checks when appropriate.						

*SD ORT = Staff Development Orientation **NE = If Not Evaluated, indicate explanation

Figure 6.2

Competency-based orientation checklist (cont.)

14. Performs BGT.							
15. Other.							
II. Communication							
A. Documents on the following forms: • Initial Interdisciplinary Assessment							
• Graphic Record							
• Interdisciplinary Progress Record							
• Nursing Discharge/ Patient Teaching							
• Interdisciplinary Plan of Care							
• Unusual Occurrence							
B. Transcribes physician's orders.							
C. Takes verbal orders from physician.							
D. Uses correct lines of communication.							
E. Attends Computer Class							
F. Gives prompt, accurate, and pertinent shift report.							
G. Interacts with patients significant others and health team members in positive manner.							

*SD ORT = Staff Development Orientation **NE = If Not Evaluated, indicate explanation

Using your skills checklists

Figure 6.2

Competency-based orientation checklist (cont.)

III. Accountability/Leadership							
A. Completes orientation statement of agreement.							
B. Delegates patient care to other personnel appropriately.							
C. Follows appropriate employee policies and procedures, i.e. call off, time off, LOA, etc.							
D. Conforms to dress code.							
E. Identifies role of the nurse in quality assurance.							
F. Maintains safe working environment.							
G. Contains costs through proper use of supplies and maintenance of equipment.							
IV. Other							
A. Has completed Human Resource/Safety Orientation							

*SD ORT = Staff Development Orientation **NE = If Not Evaluated, indicate explanation

Evidence-Based Competency Management for the Medical-Surgical Unit, Second Edition

Chapter 6

Figure 6.2

Competency-based orientation checklist (cont.)

RELEASE FROM ORIENTATION

The undersigned employee/orientee can be released from orientation as of _____ (date).

_____   _____   _____
Orientee Signature   Preceptor Signature   Unit Manager Signature

Return this form and orientation paperwork/folder to ACH Nursing Records or STH Human Resources when completed.

Skills still needing supervision are listed below. It is the responsibility of the employee/orientee to be supervised prior to performing these skills: _____
_____
_____

*SD ORT = Staff Development Orientation **NE = If Not Evaluated, indicate explanation

Source: Summa Health System Hospitals, Akron, OH. Reprinted with permission.

Using your skills checklists

Figure 6.3

Nursing assistant orientation checklist

SUMMA HEALTH SYSTEM HOSPITALS
STAFF DEVELOPMENT

COMPETENCY-BASED CHECKLIST

NURSING ASSISTANT ORIENTATION NAME: _____
SKILLS ASSESSMENT/EVALUATION HIRE DATE (this role): _____
UNIT: _____

STAFF DEVELOPMENT: INITIALS: PRECEPTORS: INITIALS:
_____   _____   _____ _____
_____   _____   _____ _____
_____   _____   _____ _____

Directions:

Orientee: Complete the self-assessment by placing a check (✓) in the appropriate column based on your level of familiarity or experience with each competency.

Staff Development/Preceptor: Complete the evaluation section for each competency after the orientee has demonstrated successful completion of that competency. Place the date and your initials in the appropriate column. If NE (not evaluated) is checked, include an explanation in the comments column.

	SELF-ASSESSMENT			EVALUATION			
Competencies	Comfortable	Need Review	Have never done	*SD ORT	Unit	**NE	Comments
A. Demonstrates ability to do basic patient care as follows:							
1. Complete bed bath							
2. Partial bath							
3. Assists with shower							
4. Oral hygiene							

*SD ORT = Staff Development Orientation **NE = If Not Evaluated, indicate explanation

Evidence-Based Competency Management for the Medical-Surgical Unit, Second Edition   105

Chapter 6

Figure 6.3

Nursing assistant orientation checklist (cont.)

5. Back care						
6. Peri care						
7. Hair care						
8. Offering/removal of bed pan/urinal						
9. Cath care						
10. Documentation of output on Kardex or worksheet						Unit based competency on file.
11. Feeding of patient, including compensatory strategies for feeding dysphagic patient						
12. Shaving of patient						
13. Occupied bed						
14. Unoccupied bed						
15. Accurately measuring patient intake and output and recording on appropriate form						
16. Patient transfer/discharge						
17. Pneumatic Cuffs						
18. K-Pad						
B. Body mechanics						
1. Discusses the proper techniques of lifting/turning/transferring patient						
2. Demonstrates proper technique in transferring patient from bed to cart and back						

*SD ORT = Staff Development Orientation **NE = If Not Evaluated, indicate explanation

Figure 6.3

Nursing assistant orientation checklist (cont.)

3. Demonstrates proper technique transferring patient from bed to wheelchair						
4. Demonstrates proper technique in positioning and turning patients						
C. Technical skills 1. Assesses patient safety including proper utilization and documentation of restraints						
2. Completes American Heart Association guidelines for Heartsaver Course						
3. Monitors oxygen tank gauge						
4. Identifies responsibilities in emergency situations						
5. Incorporates measures to reduce and prevent the spread of infection in daily patient care						
D. Demonstrates ability to take and record vital signs.						Unit based competency checklist on file.
Temperature: 1. Takes oral temperature and records						
2. Discusses procedure for rectal temperature						

*SD ORT = Staff Development Orientation **NE = If Not Evaluated, indicate explanation

Chapter 6

Figure 6.3

Nursing assistant orientation checklist (cont.)

Radial pulse: 1. Counts and records pulse rate						
Respirations: 1. Counts respiratory rate and records						
E. Demonstrates ability to obtain and transport appropriately the following specimens: 1. Sputum						
2. Urine/routine/ccms						
3. Stool						
4. Blood, transport only						
F. Performs postmortem care						
G. Transports patient to morgue						
H. Removes dirty linen or equipment from patient room						
I. Passes and picks up trays						
1. Records intake (and output) accurately on worksheet in room.						Unit based competency checklist on file.
2. Empty and replace trash bags, remove excess linen, etc., from patient rooms						

*SD ORT = Staff Development Orientation **NE = If Not Evaluated, indicate explanation

Figure 6.3

Nursing assistant orientation checklist (cont.)

K. Maintenance needs							
1. Verbalizes safety issues with equipment (step ladders, hand tools, light bulbs, etc.)							
2. Identifies light maintenance duties							
L. Demonstrates ability to Assess Just-In-Time technician. (Distribution)							
M. Demonstrates proper use of communication 1. Patient intercom							Unit based competency checklist on file.
2. Answering patient call light							
3. Telephone/answering phone appropriately by identifying unit, name, and status							
4. Operating pneumatic tube system, describe purpose and use							
5. Explaining the importance of patient confidentiality							
6. Communicating to RN any unusual observations (signs and symptoms)							
N. Interacts with patients, significant others, and health team members in positive manner.							

*SD ORT = Staff Development Orientation **NE = If Not Evaluated, indicate explanation

Evidence-Based Competency Management for the Medical-Surgical Unit, Second Edition

Figure 6.3

Nursing assistant orientation checklist (cont.)

O. Safety issues (Each orientee should be able to discuss and correctly answer questions on the following safety topics)						
1. Fire safety (Code Red)						
2. Bomb threat (Code Black)						
3. Code violet						
4. Infection prevention and exposure control						
5. Disaster (Code yellow)						
6. Evacuation						
7. Back safety						
8. Severe weather						
9. Electrical safety						
10. Code Adam						
P. Punctuality 1. Arrives on unit in uniform on time						
2. Notifies nursing office of absence according to policy						
3. Notifies nursing office of lateness according to policy						
4. Notifies nurse in charge when leaving unit and reason						

*SD ORT = Staff Development Orientation **NE = If Not Evaluated, indicate explanation

Using your skills checklists

Figure 6.3

Nursing assistant orientation checklist (cont.)

5. Follows current hospital guidelines for breaks and lunch hours							
6. Returns from errands and meetings promptly							
Q. Examinations Completes the following exams with a minimum score of 70%:							
1. Medical Abbreviation Test							
2. Patient Safety Test							
3. Patient Limited Activity Test							
4. Grooming and Oral Hygiene Test							
R. Other:							

*SD ORT = Staff Development Orientation **NE = If Not Evaluated, indicate explanation

Source: Summa Health System Hospitals, Akron, OH. Reprinted with permission.

Chapter 6

Skills checklists for annual competency assessment

This section provides suggestions on how to determine what skills to evaluate, develop the skills checklists, identify who can complete the checklists, and keep track of who has been evaluated. It also reviews what happens if someone does not meet identified competencies, and it includes a brief discussion of other methods of validating competence.

Determining what skills to evaluate

Your organization needs to set up a system to determine which competencies to evaluate each year. Chapter 2 provided a suggested formula to use when determining which skills to evaluate. There is no right or wrong way to select what skills will be evaluated, as long as the organization can justify why the particular skills were chosen. Skills should be selected based on the individual needs of the unit or organization.

Developing the skills checklists

Once the skills to be assessed are selected, skills checklists can be developed or modified from the samples attached to ensure consistency in evaluation. Review your institution's policies and procedures using current literature for support. The essential steps of the policies and procedures are incorporated into the skills checklists, many of which you can easily adapt for your institution by changing the criteria to be consistent with steps in your policies and procedures or standards.

Identifying who can complete the checklists

It is important to identify who (e.g., what job classification) can validate skills for each job classification. It may be better to have an RN or licensed practical nurse check off an NA on vital signs rather than to have another NA complete the skills checklist. Individuals who are responsible for validating someone's skill should be qualified based on education, experience, or expertise with that skill, or they should have already demonstrated proficiency with that skill. An individual with documented competence in that skill should assess ongoing competence. That competence may be determined by his or her role (e.g., advanced practice nurse, staff development instructor, unit managers, specialist coordinator, etc.), frequency of performing the skill, or already having demonstrated competence in that skill.

When introducing new technology or procedures into the clinical area, the initial training should be done by individuals with documented experience in that procedure (e.g., physicians, nurses from that specialty, vendor representatives, etc.). A core group of staff members or a single individual can be trained and can confirm the competency of other staff members after they personally demonstrate competence in that skill.

Keeping track of who has been evaluated

Each evaluator should refer to the skills checklist when observing a staff member perform that skill. Skills checklists for the competencies being evaluated can be kept in a competency notebook as a reference for the staff. These checklists can be used to assess initial and ongoing competence. The use of a checklist ensures consistency in evaluating the steps to perform the skill. Rather than completing an individual skills checklist for every person evaluated, a tracking sheet can usually be used to document completion of that skill.

The tracking sheet provides a way to document that staff members in each classification have completed required competencies. Names of the unit personnel are written on the tracking sheet, and when someone is checked off on a particular competency, the individual observing that person writes in the date and his or her initials in the column for that particular competency in the row with that person's name. Individuals are responsible for ensuring that someone validates their required skills each year. The manager then uses this information when completing performance appraisals.

The Competencies Analyzer

Figure 6.4 provides a sample tracking sheet. We've also provided an electronic version of this Excel spreadsheet on your accompanying CD-ROM. The Competencies Analyzer is an easy way for a manager to track competency assessment on his or her unit.

Figure 6.4

Competencies tracking sheet

SUMMA HEALTH SYSTEM HOSPITALS
UNIT BASED COMPETENCY CHECKLIST
Unit Secretary

MEDICAL SURGICAL UNIT: _____

EMPLOYEE NAME	COMPETENCY VERIFIED									
	SUMMA	DEPT	DIVISION	UNIT BASED						
	1. Mandatory Safety Education	2. Heart Saver	See schedule for Mandatory Ed. and SLPs							

Source: Summa Health System Hospitals, Akron, OH. Reprinted with permission.

Determining what happens when a staff member cannot perform competencies

Organizations need to identify the consequences when a staff member cannot demonstrate mastery of a competency. Policies may vary, but a mechanism needs to be in place to safeguard patients and ensure that the staff member is not assigned to a patient who requires that competency. Possible options would be to provide remediation and further clinical experiences, or to transfer the staff member to another area where he or she can meet the required competencies. Continued failure to demonstrate required competencies may lead to a plan for improvement or termination.

Other methods to validate competence

It is also important to realize that the skills checklists are only one method to validate competence; other methods may be used. Some skills may not happen frequently enough to check all staff members off on that skill, and skills fairs may be an alternative approach. During skills fairs, employees are tested and validated on skills using simulations, games, word puzzles, or other methods to verify that they are aware of the steps of the procedure. Skills checklists can also be used during fairs for those skills that may not come up frequently enough to check everyone on a unit.

With the increasing sophistication of technology, computer-assisted video evaluation may be used to evaluate competency in a particular area. Videotaped or simulated scenarios can give evaluators the opportunity to observe and rate performances. With this approach, ratings can be compared with the instructor to clarify any discrepancies and determine inter-rater reliability. However, this may not be realistic in organizations where many staff members will be completing skills checklists for their peers.

One problem with skills checklists is that you don't know whether the observed behavior is persistent and representative of the situation being observed, or whether the individual is going through the correct steps knowing that someone is evaluating him or her for that single occurrence. Therefore, indirect observation can also be used. Often, managers or charge nurses conduct patient rounds and medical record reviews. With indirect observation, there may not be direct observation of the skills, but there is the presumption that the skills are correctly followed when the desired outcomes are achieved. Clinical rounds can measure competencies as well as improve the standard of care and practice in the clinical setting.

Chapter 6

Organizations need to have a competency-based program in place to ensure that individuals are prepared to deliver quality patient care. Assessment of competency begins with orientation and continues throughout employment. An evaluation of each nursing staff member's competency should be conducted at defined intervals throughout the individual's association with the organization. Performance appraisals and skills checklists may be used to measure the ongoing competency of nursing employees. Continuing education programs and inservices can also enhance staff members' competency.

Competence assessment for the nursing staff and volunteers who provide direct patient care is based on the following:

- Populations served, including age ranges and specialties

- Competencies required for role and provision of care

- Competencies assessed during orientation

- Unit-specific competencies that need to be assessed or reassessed on a yearly basis based on care modalities, age ranges, techniques, procedures, technology, equipment, skills needed, or changes in laws and regulations

- Appropriate assessment methods for the skill being assessed

- Delineation of who is qualified to assess competence

- A description of action taken when improvement activities lead to a determination that a staff member with performance problems is unable or unwilling to improve

Individuals who transfer from another area in the organization know what competencies they must meet at the time of their orientation.

Here is a list of some questions to consider in an evaluation of the competence assessment system (Cooper 2002):

- Is new-employee competence assessment completed during the initial orientation process?

- Is employee orientation based on assessed competencies and the knowledge and skills required to deliver patient-care services?

- Is new-employee competence assessment completed at the conclusion of the orientation process?

- Do clinical staff members participate in ongoing educational activities to acquire new competencies that support patient-care delivery? Are those activities minimally based on quality improvement findings, new technology, therapeutic or pharmacology interventions, and the learning needs of the nursing staff?

- Does the management or leadership staff participate in competence assessment activities (i.e., clinical knowledge, skills, or technology)?

- Does the management or leadership staff participate in ongoing education activities to acquire new competencies for patient-care management (i.e., management development)?

- Does the performance evaluation system address staff competence?

- When competency deficiencies are noted, is a plan for correction initiated and implemented?

- Does reassessment of competence occur as necessary?

- Are summaries of competence assessment findings available by individual, by patient-care unit, and by department?

- Are plans for competence maintenance and improvement documented?

- Is an annual report submitted to the governing body?

- Do policies and procedures exist to define the process of competence assessment?

The overall competence assessment process must be reviewed on an ongoing basis to determine its effectiveness and any opportunities for improvement. This evaluation identifies what works, what doesn't, why it doesn't, and how it can be improved. It can take a very formal approach through survey methodology and interviews, or a less formal approach of asking for subjective data and feedback from key people and groups.

REFERENCES

1. Joint Commission Resources. (2008). *Comprehensive Accreditation Manual for Hospitals: The Official Handbook*. Oakbrook, IL: Joint Commission Resources.

2. Cooper, D. (2002). "The 'C' Word: Competency" in Kristen L. O'Shea, *Staff Development Nursing Secrets*. Philadelphia: Hanley & Belfus.

ALL

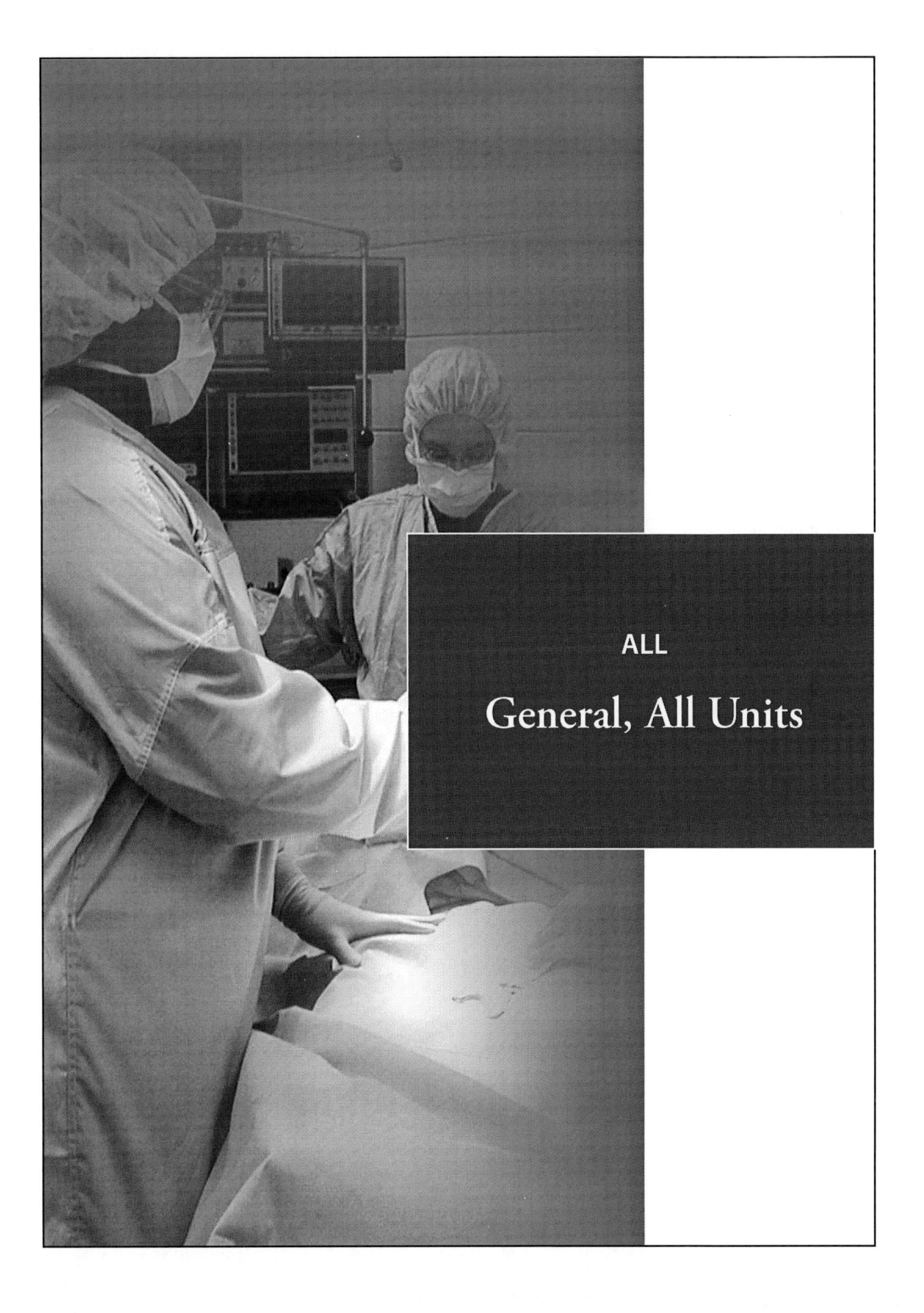

General, All Units

Contents

ABG Interpretation	121
Annual Competency Performance—Quality of Instruction	122
Arjo Ceiling Lift	123
Assessment/Validation of Competencies	124
Assisting an Adult with Feeding	125
Blood Glucose Meter	127
Blood Pressure Measurement—Automatic	129
Blood Pressure Measurement—Manual	130
Diagnostic Cardiology—Digital Holter Hook-up	132
Emergency Preparedness	133
Falls Prevention—Get Up and Go	135
Fit Testing for N-95 Respirator Masks	136
Intake and Output	137
Medication Administration	138
Oxygen Administration	140
Presentation Skills	141
Regulating and Maintaining Proper IV Rate	142
Service Excellence/Patient Satisfaction	143
Thrombolytic Therapy	144
Thrombus: Chronic versus Acute	146
Use of Automated External Defibrillator (Heartstream FR2)	147
Venipuncture with Winged Needle	148

ALL (General, All Units)

Name: _____ Date: _____

Skill: ABG Interpretation

Steps	Completed	Comments
1. Verbalizes normal ABG values 　　pH 　　pCO$_2$ 　　pO$_2$ 　　HCO$_3$		
2. Using available assessment and laboratory data, accurately determines patient's acid/base status. 　• Normal 　• Respiratory Acidosis 　• Respiratory Alkalosis 　• Metabolic Acidosis 　• Metabolic Alkalosis 　• Mixed Respiratory/Metabolic Acidosis or 　• Alkalosis		
3. Identifies at least one physical sign and/or symptom associated with the patient's ABG interpretation.		
4. Identifies at least one intervention to assist the patient in returning to a normal acid/base balance.		
5. Makes appropriate referral to physician or respiratory therapist as indicated by AFB findings.		

Self-assessment	Evaluation/ validation methods	Levels	Type of validation	Comments
❏ Experienced ❏ Need practice ❏ Never done ❏ Not applicable 　(based on scope of practice)	❏ Verbal ❏ Demonstration/ 　observation ❏ Practical exercise ❏ Interactive class	❏ Beginner ❏ Intermediate ❏ Expert	❏ Orientation ❏ Annual ❏ Other _____	

_____ _____

Employee signature　　　　　　　　　　　　　　　*Observer signature*

Reference:
Urdern, LD: Stacy, KM and Lough, ME, eds (2006). Thelan's Critical Care Nursing: Diagnosis and Management, 5th Ed. Mosby Elsevier, St. Louis, MO. P604-606.

Evidence-Based Competency Management for the Medical-Surgical Unit, Second Edition

ALL (General, All Units)

Name: _____ Date: _____

Skill: Annual Competency Performance—Quality of Instruction

Steps	Completed	Comments
1. Develops objectives that are relevant, realistic and measurable.		
2. Incorporates teaching/learning strategies to address identified needs and goals.		
3. Uses up-to-date accurate resources/materials in presentation.		
4. Picks up on verbal and nonverbal cues during session.		
5. Ensures any handouts are easily read, free of errors, and attractively designed.		
6. Bases audiovisuals on the size of the group, setting and equipment available.		
7. Provides pertinent information useful to practice.		

Self-assessment	Evaluation/ validation methods	Levels	Type of validation	Comments
❏ Experienced ❏ Need practice ❏ Never done ❏ Not applicable (based on scope of practice)	❏ Verbal ❏ Demonstration/ observation ❏ Practical exercise ❏ Interactive class	❏ Beginner ❏ Intermediate ❏ Expert	❏ Orientation ❏ Annual ❏ Other _____	

_____ _____
Employee signature   *Observer signature*

Reference:
Brunt, B. 2007. *Competencies for Staff Educators: Tools to Evaluate and Enhance Nursing Professional Development.* Marblehead, MA: HCPro, Inc.

ALL (General, All Units)

Name: _____ Date: _____

Skill: Arjo Ceiling Lift

Steps	Completed	Comments
1. Assures motor is in "charge" position when unit not in use.		
2. Identifies location and purpose of operational light indicator.		
3. Identifies red cord and explains its purpose.		

4. Uses handset to:
   a. Move lift motor off charger to desired position
   b. Lower and raise carry bar
   c. Move lift motor back to charger		

5. Demonstrates correct position of bed patient in sling and moves patient to chair
   a. Wraps sling legs properly
   b. Attaches sling loops to hook-up points on carry bar
   c. Stabilizes carry bar and patient while moving patient up and over to chair
   d. Lowers patient to chair
   e. Detaches sling from carry bar		

6. Returns unit to charge position using battery icon on handset.		
7. Locates manual operations wrench (Allen wrench) and its insertion point.		
8. Demonstrates manual operation of carry bar busing the Allen wrench.		
9. Verbalized how to clean cover of carry bar.		

Self-assessment	Evaluation/ validation methods	Levels	Type of validation	Comments
❏ Experienced ❏ Need practice ❏ Never done ❏ Not applicable (based on scope of practice)	❏ Verbal ❏ Demonstration/ observation ❏ Practical exercise ❏ Interactive class	❏ Beginner ❏ Intermediate ❏ Expert	❏ Orientation ❏ Annual ❏ Other _____	

_____   _____
Employee signature   *Observer signature*

Reference:
Doloresco, L., Lloyd, T., Smith, L., and Weinel, D. 2002. A clinical evaluation of ceiling lifts: Lifting and transfer technology for the future. *SCI Nurse* 19(2): 75-77.

Evidence-Based Competency Management for the Medical-Surgical Unit, Second Edition

ALL (General, All Units)

Name: _____ Date: _____

Skill: **Assessment/Validation of Competencies**

Steps	Completed	Comments
1. Demonstrates proficiency in skill being validated.		
2. Uses appropriate validation method(s).		
3. Validates performance according to established standards, e.g., checklist.		
4. Provides appropriate feedback to learner.		
5. Documents competency on appropriate form(s).		

Self-assessment	Evaluation/ validation methods	Levels	Type of validation	Comments
❏ Experienced ❏ Need practice ❏ Never done ❏ Not applicable (based on scope of practice)	❏ Verbal ❏ Demonstration/ observation ❏ Practical exercise ❏ Interactive class	❏ Beginner ❏ Intermediate ❏ Expert	❏ Orientation ❏ Annual ❏ Other _____	

_____   _____
Employee signature   *Observer signature*

Reference:
Brunt, B. 2007. *Competencies for Staff Educators: Tools to Evaluate and Enhance Nursing Professional Development.* Marblehead, MA: HCPro, Inc.

ALL (General, All Units)

Name: _____ Date: _____

Skill: Assisting an Adult with Feeding

Steps	Completed	Comments
1. Removes distasteful sights & odors from room, provides adequate ventilation, and clean surroundings for mealtime.		
2. Offers patient hand cleansing with a warm wash cloth & soap, or disinfecting gel.		
3. Positions patient comfortably upright in a chair, if possible. • Consults ST/RN/MD for best positioning of patient if unable to get into chair.		
4. Washes hands and brings tray to area.		
5. Verifies that the patient has the correct diet on tray, checks armband; asks patient to verify name, and doctor, or other identifying data.		
6. Ensures that diet is correct in PLATO, agrees with ST recommendations.		
7. Ensures food is the correct temperature and that liquids are thickened as ordered. Rewarms food and/or thickens liquids as needed.		
8. Prepares food, if necessary, by opening cartons, buttering bread, and cutting meat.		
9. Identifies foods, & describes location to patient.		
10. Drapes patient with towel or napkins.		
11. Sits in a comfortable position to feed the patient.		
12. Offers the patient small amounts of food at a time. Offers liquids as requested or between bites. • Follows speech therapist guidelines, i.e., positioning chin down towards chest when swallowing, or other positions to assist the patient as ordered.		
13. Lets the patient choose what he or she would like to eat next, unless directed by ST order.		
14. Warns patient about hot food and waits for it to cool.		
15. Does not rush the patient. Allows patient to chew and swallow the food before offering more. Uses a spoon to feed patient.		

Evidence-Based Competency Management for the Medical-Surgical Unit, Second Edition

ALL (General, All Units)

• If new swallowing problems are observed, refers patient immediately for Bedside Swallow screening by RN, or ST per unit protocol.		
16. Encourages patient to hold bread or toast and to feed self when possible.		
17. Wipes the patient's mouth and chin when necessary.		
18. Allows for rest periods for the patient who tires easily.		
19. Moves the tray away from the patient.		
20. Checks the patient's gown and bed for spillage of food.		
21. Replaces any items removed from the bedside table (call light, telephone, urinal, Kleenex, etc.).		
22. Offers mouth care and hand washing after eating.		
23. Repositions the patient comfortably. • If at risk for aspiration, has the head of bed elevated for 30 minutes after eating and follows ST guidelines.		
24. Records fluids on I&O record on the door.		
25. Records percentage of meal eaten in patient record on PLATO.		
26. If patient on a calorie count, unit may collect Menus for calorie count in envelope on door.		

Self-assessment	Evaluation/ validation methods	Levels	Type of validation	Comments
❏ Experienced ❏ Need practice ❏ Never done ❏ Not applicable (based on scope of practice)	❏ Verbal ❏ Demonstration/ observation ❏ Practical exercise ❏ Interactive class	❏ Beginner ❏ Intermediate ❏ Expert	❏ Orientation ❏ Annual ❏ Other _____	

_____   _____
Employee signature   *Observer signature*

Reference:
Perry, A. and Potter, P. 2006. *Clinical Nursing Skills & Techniques.* 6th Ed. St. Louis, MO: Mosby.

ALL (General, All Units)

Name: _____ Date: _____

Skill: Blood Glucose Meter

Steps	Completed	Comments
1. Demonstrates how to properly clean meter.		
2. Turns on meter and correctly verifies test strip code.		
3. Performs check strip validation correctly.		
4. Performs high & low controls according to instructions/prompts.		
5. Explains or demonstrates how to appropriately document quality control (QC) results (QC log).		
6. Explains or demonstrates how to correct a "failed" QC result.		
7. Explains/demonstrates how to document the corrective action on a "failed" QC result.		
Patient testing		
1. Properly identifies patient.		
2. Describes procedure to patient.		
3. Wears appropriate personal protective equipment (PPE) when collecting/handling sample.		
4. Assesses patient's fingertips and chooses appropriate site for sample collection.		
5. Explains or demonstrates purpose of test code chip and how to replace.		
6. Turns on meter and verifies test strip code correctly.		
7. Correctly inserts test strip into meter.		
8. Correctly obtains blood sample from fingerstick.		
9. Applies sufficient amount of blood sample to test strip.		
10. Documents patient result on appropriate form/chart.		
11. Provides appropriate postfingerstick care to patient.		
12. Discards testing materials in appropriate containers (i.e., lancet, test strip, etc.).		

Evidence-Based Competency Management for the Medical-Surgical Unit, Second Edition

ALL (General, All Units)

13. States critical value ranges when a sample is to be collected and sent to the laboratory for analysis.		
14. Explains or demonstrates the collection of a confirmation sample.		
15. Reviewed current procedure for relevant revisions.		

Self-assessment	Evaluation/ validation methods	Levels	Type of validation	Comments
❏ Experienced ❏ Need practice ❏ Never done ❏ Not applicable (based on scope of practice)	❏ Verbal ❏ Demonstration/ observation ❏ Practical exercise ❏ Interactive class	❏ Beginner ❏ Intermediate ❏ Expert	❏ Orientation ❏ Annual ❏ Other _____	

_____ _____
Employee signature *Observer signature*

Reference:
Duell, D., Martin, B., and Smith, S. 2008. *Clinical Nursing Skills: Basic to Advanced Skills*. 7th ed. Upper Saddle River, NJ: Pearson Education, Inc.

ALL (General, All Units)

Name: _____ Date: _____

Skill: Blood Pressure Measurement—Automatic

Steps	Completed	Comments
1. Identifies patient and explains procedure.		
2. Selects an appropriately sized blood-pressure cuff for the patient, attaches to machine.		
3. Locates the brachial artery (inner aspect of the elbow) and feels for pulse.		
4. Places cuff so the inflatable bag is centered over the brachial artery and the lower edge of the cuff is 1-2 inches above pulse site.		
5. Wraps cuff around the arm snugly; fastens it securely.		
6. Places patient's arm in position of comfort, relaxed at or below level of patient's heart.		
7. Turns Monitor "ON," and pushes Start button.		
8. Reads Blood Pressure accurately and reports to patient's nurse if outside expected measurement for patient, or normal range.		
9. Records measurement in PLATO or on paper graphic if PLATO is not available.		
10. Removes cuff, and places patient in position of comfort and safety.		

Self-assessment	Evaluation/ validation methods	Levels	Type of validation	Comments
❏ Experienced ❏ Need practice ❏ Never done ❏ Not applicable (based on scope of practice)	❏ Verbal ❏ Demonstration/ observation ❏ Practical exercise ❏ Interactive class	❏ Beginner ❏ Intermediate ❏ Expert	❏ Orientation ❏ Annual ❏ Other _____	

_____   _____
Employee signature   *Observer signature*

Reference:
Duell, D., Martin, B., and Smith, S. 2008. *Clinical Nursing Skills: Basic to Advanced Skills.* 7th ed. Upper Saddle River, NJ: Pearson Education, Inc.

Evidence-Based Competency Management for the Medical-Surgical Unit, Second Edition

ALL (General, All Units)

Name: _____ Date: _____

Skill: Blood Pressure Measurement—Manual

Steps	Completed	Comments
1. Identifies patient and explains procedure.		
2. Selects an appropriately sized blood-pressure cuff for the patient.		
3. Locates the brachial artery (inner aspect of the elbow).		
4. Places cuff so the inflatable bag is centered over the brachial artery and the lower edge of the cuff is about one to two inches above site.		
5. Wraps cuff around the arm snugly; fastens it securely or tucks the end of the cuff well under the preceding wrapping.		
6. Places the stethoscope into ears and closes the screw valve on the air pump.		
7. With the fingertips of left hand, feels for the pulse over brachial artery. Places stethoscope firmly but with little pressure over area.		
8. Palpates brachial artery with left hand and pumps bulb until gauge rises about 30 mmHg above the point at which the brachial pulse disappears, or pumps bulb until gauge is 30 mmHg above the point that the BP has been running.		
9. Uses the valve on the bulb to release air slowly, and notes the point on the manometer at which the first of two consecutive beats is heard (systolic pressure).		
10. Continues to release air in the cuff evenly and slowly. Notes the reading on the manometer when all sounds disappear (diastolic pressure).		
11. Allows the remaining air to escape quickly and removes the cuff.		
12. Documents blood pressure reading on graphic record.		

ALL (General, All Units)

Self-assessment	Evaluation/ validation methods	Levels	Type of validation	Comments
❏ Experienced ❏ Need practice ❏ Never done ❏ Not applicable (based on scope of practice)	❏ Verbal ❏ Demonstration/ observation ❏ Practical exercise ❏ Interactive class	❏ Beginner ❏ Intermediate ❏ Expert	❏ Orientation ❏ Annual ❏ Other _____	

_____

Employee signature

_____

Observer signature

Reference:
Duell, D., Martin, B., and Smith, S. 2008. *Clinical Nursing Skills: Basic to Advanced Skills*. 7th ed. Upper Saddle River, NJ: Pearson Education, Inc.

ALL (General, All Units)

Name: _____ Date: _____

Skill: Diagnostic Cardiology—Digital Holter Hook-up

Steps	Completed	Comments
UPLOADING STUDIES		
1. Demonstrate verification of patient recording (serial number or diary return).		
2. Demonstrate use of Load screen…logging appropriate information.		
3. Demonstrate physical connection to computer.		
4. Demonstrate send to out-box function.		
5. Demonstrate removal of battery.		
6. Demonstrate proper cleaning of recorder and cable.		
DOWNLOADING REPORTS		
1. Demonstrate understanding and navigation between in-box and archive.		
2. Demonstrate retrieval from in-box to view.		
3. Demonstrate view and print reverse order functions.		
4. Demonstrate move from in-box to archive function.		
5. Demonstrate reconciliation between charts and reports.		
6. Demonstrate reconciliation between reports and recorders.		

Self-assessment	Evaluation/ validation methods	Levels	Type of validation	Comments
❏ Experienced ❏ Need practice ❏ Never done ❏ Not applicable (based on scope of practice)	❏ Verbal ❏ Demonstration/ observation ❏ Practical exercise ❏ Interactive class	❏ Beginner ❏ Intermediate ❏ Expert	❏ Orientation ❏ Annual ❏ Other _____	

_____   _____
Employee signature   *Observer signature*

Reference:
Nissen, S., Pepine, C., Bashore, T., et al. 1994. American College of Cardiology position statement. Cardiac angiography without cine film: erecting a "tower of Babel" in the cardiac catheterization laboratory. *Journal of the American College of Cardiology* 24: 834-837.

Name: _____ Date: _____

Skill: Emergency Preparedness

Steps	Completed	Comments
1. Assesses if a medical emergency exists: physical assessment (patient responsiveness, LOC, vitals); historical assessment (diabetes, autonomic neuropathy, hypotensive episodes).		
2. Identifies correct pathway cardiac rehab emergency treatment algorithm.		
3. Demonstrates ventilation technique via Resusci mask.		
4. Demonstrates O^2 to ambu bag and nasal cannula hook-up.		
5. Demonstrates fitting patient with nasal cannula.		
6. Performs BLS ABCs and one cycle of rescue breathing and cardiac compressions.		
7. Identifies team code number to call.		
8. Demonstrates technique for transferring patient from telemetry to defibrillator leads, selects limb and augmented lead positions, runs an ECG strip.		
9. Transports team cart and gurney from exam room to exercise area.		
10. Identifies team cart components: emergency drug box, phase IV solutions, IV start sets, pulse oximeter.		
11. Demonstrates: placement of conductive defib pads on the chest wall, placement and pressure on the defib paddles, and the correct sequence of ACLS defibrillation shocks.		
12. Demonstrates technique for transferring patient to gurney and transporting patient to exam room or ED.		

ALL (General, All Units)

Self-assessment	Evaluation/ validation methods	Levels	Type of validation	Comments
❏ Experienced ❏ Need practice ❏ Never done ❏ Not applicable (based on scope of practice)	❏ Verbal ❏ Demonstration/ observation ❏ Practical exercise ❏ Interactive class	❏ Beginner ❏ Intermediate ❏ Expert	❏ Orientation ❏ Annual ❏ Other _____	

_____

Employee signature

_____

Observer signature

Reference:
Gazmuri, R. et al. 2007. Scientific knowledge gaps and clinical research priorities for cardiopulmonary resuscitation and emergency cardiac care identified during the 2005 international consensus conference on E and CPR science with treatment recommendations: A consensus statement from the International Liaison Committee on Resuscitation, the American Heart Association Emergency Cardiovascular Care Committee, the Stroke Council and Cardiovascular Nursing Council. *Circulation* 116: 2501-2512.

ALL (General, All Units)

Name: _____ Date: _____

Skill: Falls Prevention—Get Up and Go

Steps	Completed	Comments
1. Verbalize three factors related to hospitalization which increase the risk of falls for elderly in the hospital.		

2. Demonstrate the steps of the Get Up and Go Test, as if the patient.
   a. Have the patient sit in a chair
   b. Instruct the patient to stand up
   c. Ask the patient to stand still with eyes open
   d. Ask patient to close eyes and stand still
   e. Instruct patient to open eyes and walk 10 feet, turn around and come back
   f. Ask patient to sit down in the chair again		

3. Verbalize at least one factor to assess during each step of the testing.		

4. Differentiate the timed results of the test as to risk for falls. Be able to state:
   a. Less than 20 seconds is low risk
   b. 20-30 seconds moderate risk
   c. Greater than 30 seconds is high risk		

5. List at least 5 nursing interventions for falls prevention.		

Self-assessment	Evaluation/ validation methods	Levels	Type of validation	Comments
❏ Experienced ❏ Need practice ❏ Never done ❏ Not applicable (based on scope of practice)	❏ Verbal ❏ Demonstration/ observation ❏ Practical exercise ❏ Interactive class	❏ Beginner ❏ Intermediate ❏ Expert	❏ Orientation ❏ Annual ❏ Other _____	

_____ _____
Employee signature   ***Observer signature***

Reference:
American Geriatrics Society, British Geriatrics Society, and American Academy of Orthopaedic Surgeons Panel on Falls Prevention. 2001. Guidelines for the prevention of falls in older persons. *Journal of the American Geriatrics Society* 49(5): 664-672.

ALL (General, All Units)

Name: _____ Date: _____

Skill: Fit Testing for N-95 Respirator Masks

Steps	Completed	Comments
1. Identifies if the employee has completed the Respiratory Questionnaire. Notes what (if any) answers on the questionnaire would indicate the employee should not be Fit Tested. (Based on the OSHA Respiratory Protection Standards.)		
2. Explains the Fit Test Procedure to the employee.		
3. Performs the Fit test per the OSHA Respiratory Protection Standards. Performs a Sensitivity Check on the employee with either saccharin solution or bitrex solution. Appropriately uses bitrex solution if the employee cannot taste the saccharin solution. Assists the employee to put on the N-95 respirator mask, coaching the employee on assuring a good tight fit and how to adjust the mask as appropriate. Performs the Fit Test on the employee (noting each step that should be carried out during the testing process – regular breathing, deep breathing, turning head from side to side, nodding up and down, talking, grimacing and frowning, and smiling). Assists the employee to readjust their mask if needed during the process. Verbalizes when another mask should be used in the Fit Test procedure. Explains to the employee when to wear their mask.		

Self-assessment	Evaluation/ validation methods	Levels	Type of validation	Comments
❏ Experienced ❏ Need practice ❏ Never done ❏ Not applicable (based on scope of practice)	❏ Verbal ❏ Demonstration/ observation ❏ Practical exercise ❏ Interactive class	❏ Beginner ❏ Intermediate ❏ Expert	❏ Orientation ❏ Annual ❏ Other _____	

_____   _____
Employee signature   *Observer signature*

Reference:
United States Department of Labor Occupational Safety and Health Administration. Fit testing guidelines. Standards 29CFR 1910.134, Appendix A.

ALL (General, All Units)

Name: _____ Date: _____

Skill: Intake and Output

Steps	Completed	Comments
1. Diet: Estimates % of diet eaten from tray each meal. Records amount of taken in on door as tray is removed from room.		
2. Fluids: Identifies number of cc's taken in by patient in the form of liquids, pop, jello, or ice. Locates and uses unit reference for fluids as necessary. Documents on door slip for appropriate shift.		
3. Output: Using proper PPE empties and measures amount of urine in bedpan or urinal, or foley.		
4. Disposes of urine. Washes hands.		
5. Record amount of urine on door slip.		

Self-assessment	Evaluation/ validation methods	Levels	Type of validation	Comments
❏ Experienced ❏ Need practice ❏ Never done ❏ Not applicable (based on scope of practice)	❏ Verbal ❏ Demonstration/ observation ❏ Practical exercise ❏ Interactive class	❏ Beginner ❏ Intermediate ❏ Expert	❏ Orientation ❏ Annual ❏ Other _____	

_____   _____
Employee signature   **Observer signature**

Reference:
Alvare, S., Dugan, D., and Fuzy, J. 2005. *Nursing Assistant Care*. Albuquerque, NM: Hartman Publishing.

ALL (General, All Units)

Name: _____ Date: _____

Skill: Medication Administration

Steps	Completed	Comments
Routine Medications:		
1. Verifies all pages of the MAR/Medication Record are present. a. When giving the first dose of any medication checks for last dose given of a similar-acting medication so appropriate time interval can be maintained.		
2. Takes MAR & COW to verify and prepare medications.		
3. Identify the patient by checking the following: a. Patient name and medical record number/birthday on identification band with patient name and medical record number on MAR.		

4. **Check allergies each time a medication is administered. Identify allergies by checking:**
    a. For red allergy arm band
    b. For documentation of allergies on MAR, Home Medication List, FACT Sheet, or on History & Physical. Electronic chart utilize information tab or header.		

5. Check the label sent with pharmacy against MAR; if it does not match, a check of the order is done.		
6. Check when giving the first dose of any medication for last dose given of a similar-acting medication so appropriate time interval can be maintained.		

7. Opens unit-dose packaging at the bedside when patient is ready to take the medication. Places medication in a cup or directly in the patient's hand.
    a. Takes pill cutter or crusher to bedside **and splits or crushes medication at the bedside**.
    b. Uses appropriate syringe if patient has Dobhoff/NGT.		

8. **Stays with the patient until medication is administered and does not leave medication at bedside unless ordered.**		
9. When administering oral medications, raises the patient to a sitting position if condition permits. Gives sufficient fluid to facilitate swallowing.		
10. Sanitize hands.		
11. Documents **after** medication is given with initial.		
12. If the medication is NOT given, circles time and initials. **Indicates the reason for omission on MAR/medication record.** a. **If medication is given late, documents time med was given.**		
13. **Signs each sheet of the MAR or medication record in appropriate shift block.**		
14. **Documents fluid intake amount (IV or PO) if patient on I & O record.**		

Self-assessment	Evaluation/ validation methods	Levels	Type of validation	Comments
❏ Experienced ❏ Need practice ❏ Never done ❏ Not applicable (based on scope of practice)	❏ Verbal ❏ Demonstration/ observation ❏ Practical exercise ❏ Interactive class	❏ Beginner ❏ Intermediate ❏ Expert	❏ Orientation ❏ Annual ❏ Other _____	

_____   _____

Employee signature   **Observer signature**

Reference:
Perry, A. and Potter, P. 2006. *Clinical Nursing Skills & Techniques.* 6th Ed. St. Louis, MO: Mosby Elsevier.

ALL (General, All Units)

Name: _____ Date: _____

Skill: Oxygen Administration

Steps	Completed	Comments
1. Verifies the physician's order.		
2. Washes hands.		
3. Obtains the required equipment: 　a. Oxygen flowmeter 　b. Humidifier (over 4 liters) 　c. Sterile water (over 4 liters) 　d. Oxygen connecting tubing (if needed) 　e. Oxygen administration device		
4. Identifies the patient and explains procedure.		
5. Adjusts the device to the ordered level.		
6. Applies the device to the patient.		
7. Confirms FiO_2 as appropriate.		
8. Leaves the patient area clean and safe after disposing of excess equipment.		
9. Washes hands before leaving room.		
10. Documents equipment, concentration, or liter flow in the patient's chart.		

Self-assessment	Evaluation/ validation methods	Levels	Type of validation	Comments
❏ Experienced ❏ Need practice ❏ Never done ❏ Not applicable (based on scope of practice)	❏ Verbal ❏ Demonstration/ observation ❏ Practical exercise ❏ Interactive class	❏ Beginner ❏ Intermediate ❏ Expert	❏ Orientation ❏ Annual ❏ Other _____	

_____　　_____
Employee signature　　　　　　　　　　　　　　　*Observer signature*

Reference:
Duell, D., Martin, B., and Smith, S. 2008. *Clinical Nursing Skills: Basic to Advanced Skills.* 7th ed. New Jersey: Pearson Education, Inc.

Perry, A. and Potter, P. 2006. *Clinical Nursing Skills & Techniques.* 6th Ed. St. Louis, MO: Mosby Elsevier.

ALL (General, All Units)

Name: _____ Date: _____

Skill: Presentation Skills

Steps	Completed	Comments
1. Uses appropriate teaching methods for content being taught.		
2. Speaks clearly.		
3. Presents in organized manner.		
4. Maintains eye contact.		
5. Presents at the level of the learner.		
6. Summarizes material.		
7. Encourages audience participation.		
8. Correlates theory to practice.		
9. Generates learner questions.		
10. Gives participants opportunity to evaluate program.		
11. Administers and reviews pre- and posttests with the participants.		

Self-assessment	Evaluation/ validation methods	Levels	Type of validation	Comments
❏ Experienced ❏ Need practice ❏ Never done ❏ Not applicable (based on scope of practice)	❏ Verbal ❏ Demonstration/ observation ❏ Practical exercise ❏ Interactive class	❏ Beginner ❏ Intermediate ❏ Expert	❏ Orientation ❏ Annual ❏ Other _____	

_____   _____
Employee signature   ***Observer signature***

Reference:
Brunt, B. 2007. *Competencies for Staff Educators: Tools to Evaluate and Enhance Nursing Professional Development.* Marblehead, MA: HCPro, Inc.

Evidence-Based Competency Management for the Medical-Surgical Unit, Second Edition

ALL (General, All Units)

Name: _____ Date: _____

Skill: Regulating and Maintaining Proper IV Rate

Steps	Completed	Comments

Observations to be made during IV infusion.
  A. Initial shift assessment identifies:
     1. Correct fluid is handling.
     2. Infusing at correct rate.
     3. Verifies all pump settings are correct.
     4. All connections are intact.
     5. IV tubing off floor.
     6. No kinks in tubing.
     7. Drip chamber with correct fluid level.
     8. Dressing occlusive.
     9. IV site clear, without redness or swelling (benign).
     10. Dates on tubing/dressing of initiation.
     11. Verbalized date of site, tubing and dressing changes.		

B. Assessment to be made q1°
     1. IV running at correct rate.
     2. All pump settings correct.
     3. IV site benign.
     4. Tubing intact and without kinks.		

Self-assessment	Evaluation/ validation methods	Levels	Type of validation	Comments
❏ Experienced ❏ Need practice ❏ Never done ❏ Not applicable (based on scope of practice)	❏ Verbal ❏ Demonstration/ observation ❏ Practical exercise ❏ Interactive class	❏ Beginner ❏ Intermediate ❏ Expert	❏ Orientation ❏ Annual ❏ Other _____	

_____   _____

Employee signature   *Observer signature*

Reference:
Weinstein, S. 2007. *Plumer's Principles and Practice of Intravenous Therapy*. 8th ed. Philadelphia, PA: Lippincott.

ALL (General, All Units)

Name: _____ Date: _____

Skill: **Service Excellence/Patient Satisfaction**

Steps	Completed	Comments
Uses the "3 Cs" principles of caring, concern, and communication by following AIDET:		
1. <u>Acknowledges</u> patient by name; makes eye contact; asks "is there anything I can do for you?"		
2. <u>Introduces</u> self by name and skillset, professional certification, and experience.		
3. <u>Duration</u> gives an accurate time expectation for tests, tray delivery, and/or physician arrival.		
4. <u>Explains</u> step by step what will happen, answers questions; leaves phone number or method to reach you. Assures privacy. Connects key words with patient safety and excellent care.		
5. <u>Thanks</u> the patient for choosing Summa; expresses concern for inconvenience often caused by healthcare experience. Thanks the patient's family for assistance and support of the patient.		

Self-assessment	Evaluation/ validation methods	Levels	Type of validation	Comments
❏ Experienced ❏ Need practice ❏ Never done ❏ Not applicable (based on scope of practice)	❏ Verbal ❏ Demonstration/ observation ❏ Practical exercise ❏ Interactive class	❏ Beginner ❏ Intermediate ❏ Expert	❏ Orientation ❏ Annual ❏ Other _____	

_____ _____
Employee signature *Observer signature*

Reference:
Studer, Q. 2003. *Hardwiring Excellence*. Gulf Breeze, FL: Fire Starter Publishing.

Evidence-Based Competency Management for the Medical-Surgical Unit, Second Edition

ALL (General, All Units)

Name: _____ Date: _____

Skill: **Thrombolytic Therapy**

Steps	Completed	Comments
Before therapy is begun: 1. Established 2 vascular access sites (one may be HL) and checks sites at least q 15 min.		
2. Verbalized contraindications. (Uncontrolled hypertension, history of bleeding ulcer, active internal bleeding, recent intracranial/intraspinal surgery or trauma, intracranial neoplasm, AV malformation, aneurysm.)		
3. Uses caution/gentleness when moving patient.		
4. Obtains baseline VS and neuron status.		
5. Obtains baseline laboratory values (Hemogram, PT, PTT, fibrinogen, electrolytes, CPK).		
6. Avoids repeated needle punctures (blood draws are grouped, avoid IM injections if possible).		
During therapy infusion: 1. Monitor VS and neuron status q 15 min and notifies physician of change immediately.		
2. Checks arm under blood pressure cuff for ecchymosis q 1 hour. Rotates cuff prn.		
3. Monitor for signs of reperfusion (decreased chest pain, resolution of ST elevation, development of arrhythmias).		
4. Looks for subtle signs of bleeding (tachycardia, orthostatic hypotension).		
5. Assess all body drainage for presence of blood findings (urine/stool/emesis/gastric drainage).		
6. Monitors lab values (H&H, PT, PTT, other coag, BUN, Creat, Cardiac markers).		
7. Applies pressure to all venipuncture sites for at least 5 minutes.		
8. Identifies risk factors for clot information (elderly, diabetic, smoking hs., elevated lipids, hypertension, sedentary lifestyle).		
After therapy is completed: 1. Monitors VS and neuron check's q 15 min x 2 hr then q 1 hr x 2 then q 2 hr. x 24hrs.		

ALL (General, All Units)

2. Monitors lab values using 2nd IV site q 12 hr x 24 hr then qd x2.		
3. Assess for subtle signs of bleeding (as above) q 12 hr.		
4. Assess for signs of reocclusion and notifies physician immediately (Recurrent chest pain, ST segment elevation, diaphoresis, nausea, arrhythmia).		
5. Educates the patient about the current therapy and also the probable use of a "blood thinner" at home (Coumadin booklet).		

Self-assessment	Evaluation/ validation methods	Levels	Type of validation	Comments
❏ Experienced ❏ Need practice ❏ Never done ❏ Not applicable (based on scope of practice)	❏ Verbal ❏ Demonstration/ observation ❏ Practical exercise ❏ Interactive class	❏ Beginner ❏ Intermediate ❏ Expert	❏ Orientation ❏ Annual ❏ Other _____	

_____ _____

Employee signature **Observer signature**

Reference:
American College of Cardiology and the American Heart Association. *ACC/AHA Guideline for the Management of Patients With ST-Elevation Myocardial Infarction Pocket Guide.* 2004.

ALL (General, All Units)

Name: _____ Date: _____

Skill: **Thrombus: Chronic versus Acute**

Steps	Completed	Comments
1. Performs venous duplex study according to protocol.		
2. Reviews patient chart for previous DVT, PE history.		
3. Observes and documents for acute DVT: • Dilatation of vessel • Sonolucent echoes with difficulty compressing • No or poor spontaneous flow • Poor augmention		
4. Observes and documents for chronic DVT: • Recanalization • Heterogeneous or bright echoes • Collaterals • Small vessel or atrophy of vessel • Incompetency of valves • Patient history of previous DVT, PE		

Self-assessment	Evaluation/ validation methods	Levels	Type of validation	Comments
❏ Experienced ❏ Need practice ❏ Never done ❏ Not applicable (based on scope of practice)	❏ Verbal ❏ Demonstration/ observation ❏ Practical exercise ❏ Interactive class	❏ Beginner ❏ Intermediate ❏ Expert	❏ Orientation ❏ Annual ❏ Other _____	

_____   _____
Employee signature   *Observer signature*

Reference:
National Heart Lung and Blood Institute. 2007. *Deep vein thrombosis.* United States Department of Health and Human Services.

ALL (General, All Units)

Name: _____ Date: _____

Skill: Use of Automated External Defibrillator (Heartstream FR2)

Steps	Completed	Comments
1. Assesses the patient for unconsciousness, no breathing, and no detectable pulse.		
2. Turns on the Heartstream FR2.		
3. Simulates proper skin prep prior to pads placement.		
4. Correctly places defibrillation pads.		
5. Plugs the pads connector into Heartstream FR2's connector port.		
6. Ensures no one touches the patient when Heartstream FR2 is analyzing.		
7. Verbally and visually clears the patient prior to delivering shock.		
8. Presses shock button when advised.		
9. Assesses patient for presence of a pulse when the Heartstream FR2 gives a "No Shock Advised" message.		

Self-assessment	Evaluation/ validation methods	Levels	Type of validation	Comments
❏ Experienced ❏ Need practice ❏ Never done ❏ Not applicable (based on scope of practice)	❏ Verbal ❏ Demonstration/ observation ❏ Practical exercise ❏ Interactive class	❏ Beginner ❏ Intermediate ❏ Expert	❏ Orientation ❏ Annual ❏ Other _____	

_____   _____
Employee signature   *Observer signature*

Reference:
American Heart Association. 2005. American Heart Association guidelines for cardiopulmonary resuscitation and emergency cardiovascular care. *Circulation* 112: IV35-IV46.

ALL (General, All Units)

Name: _____   Date: _____

Skill: Venipuncture with Winged Needle

Steps	Completed	Comments
1. Washes hands.		
2. Obtains IV tray ensuring equipment is present (winged needle, prep swabs, tourniquet, dressing, and tape).		

3. Organizes and prepares:
  a. Winged needle
  b. Prep swabs (alcohol or bedadine)
  c. Tourniquet
  d. Tape
  e. Dressing
  f. Towel or disposable blue underpad
  g. Gloves		

4. Explains procedure to patient.		
5. Identifies site, stating criteria for selection (avoids bony prominences, wrist, and dominate hand and uses most distal vein).		
6. Dons gloves.		
7. Selects size winged needle and states criteria for selection.		
8. Places tourniquet 5–6" above site to obstruct venous flow only.		
9. Selects vein.		
10. Cleanses site (from center out using betadine or alcohol).		
11. Removes cap from needle.		
12. Holds hand or forearm with nondominant hand and secures vein beneath insertion site with thumb.		
13. Places needle bevel up at 30–45° angle from skin and punctures vein.		
14. Observes blood return.		
15. Advances winged needle into vein an additional one-quarter to one-half inch		
16. Releases tourniquet.		
17. Attaches IV tubing.		

18. Applies IV dressing.		
19. Tapes IV tubing.		
20. Labels IV dressing.		
21. Labels IV tubing.		
22. Removes gloves and discards.		
23. Washes hands.		
24. States appropriate number of times allowed for venipuncture, if unsuccessful, and steps to take once that number has been reached.		
25. Documents procedure.		

Self-assessment	Evaluation/ validation methods	Levels	Type of validation	Comments
❏ Experienced ❏ Need practice ❏ Never done ❏ Not applicable (based on scope of practice)	❏ Verbal ❏ Demonstration/ observation ❏ Practical exercise ❏ Interactive class	❏ Beginner ❏ Intermediate ❏ Expert	❏ Orientation ❏ Annual ❏ Other _____	

_____   _____

Employee signature   *Observer signature*

Reference:
Weinstein, S. 2007. *Plumer's Principles and Practice of Intravenous Therapy*. 8th ed. Philadelphia, PA: Lippincott.

MS
Medical-Surgical

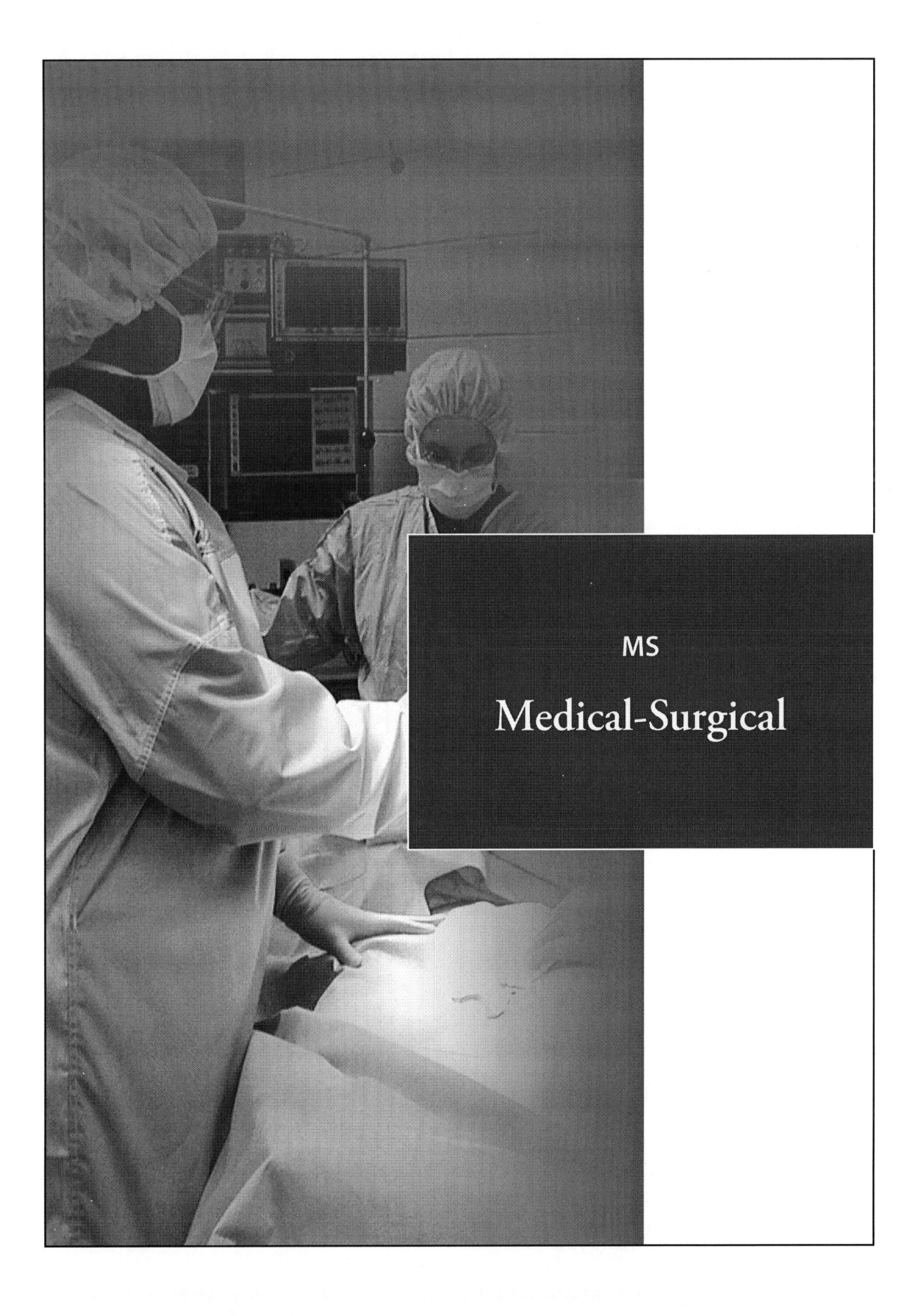

MS—Medical-Surgical

Contents

Accessing Implantable Access Devices	154
Adding IV Solution, Priming Tubing, Changing Tubing	155
Adding IV Solution to Central Line	157
Administration of Blood	158
Applanation Tonometry	161
Appointment Scheduling—Clinic	162
Atrium Ocean (Wet) Chest Tube Collection Set-Up	163
Barthel Index—Modified Rankin Scale	165
Bed Bath	166
BICAP and Cautery	168
Bladder Scan	169
Blood Culture Collection	170
Braden Scale	172
CADD Pump	173
Care of the Patient with Central Venous Catheters	175
Central Venous Catheter—Application of Sterile Occlusive Dressing	177
Central Venous Catheter—Obtaining Blood Samples	179
Central Venous Catheter—Removal	181
Chemotherapy Administration	183
Chemotherapy Teaching	185
Chest Drainage Autotransfusion—Atrium Unit	187
Chest Tube Dressing Change	189
Code Management/Med-Surg	190
Conscious Sedation	192
Conversion to Intermittent Infusion of Continuous IV	194
Crutch Walking and Use of Walker	196
Discontinuing IV Therapy	197
Drug Testing, Blood and Urine	198
Flex Pen® Patient Self-Administration	200
Gemstar Pump	202
Homegoing Instructions	206
Hypodermoclysis	208
Infusion Intravenous Piggyback Antibiotics (IVPB)	210
Inline Tracheobronchial Suctioning	212
Insertion of Dobbhoff Feeding Tube	214
Insulin Administration	216
Insulin Administration Instruction	218
Intramuscular Injections	220
Intravenous Catheters—Declotting	221
IV Dressing Changes	222
IV Site—Drawing Blood	224
IV Start—Hemodialysis Catheter	225
IV Starts and PRN Adapter	227
IV Therapy Documentation	228
Lab Specimen Labeling Compliance	230
Lidocaine for Insertion of IV Catheters	231
Maintenance of Hickman Catheter	232
Metered Dose Inhaler (MDI)	233

Nasogastric Tube Maintenance	234
Nasopharyngeal Suctioning	235
Neurological Assessment and Documentation	237
Neurovascular Status of the Spinal Unit	240
Neutropenic Precautions	241
NIH Stroke Scale, Completing the National Institutes of Health	242
Normal Saline Wet to Dry Dressing	243
Ocular Medication Administration	245
Ophthalmic Medication Administration	246
Oral Care of the Cancer Patient	248
Patient-Controlled Analgesia (PCA) Infuser	249
Peripheral Blood Draw	250
PICC Line (Applying a PRN Adapter)	252
PICC Line (Obtaining Blood Samples)	253
PICC Line (Removing the PICC)	254
PICC Line (Starting and Discontinuing an Infusion)	255
PICCS, Midlines and Central Lines—Suturing	257
Pin Care	258
Postoperative Assessment	259
Presenting a Patient at Team Rounds	261
Pulse Oximeter Monitor	263
Pyxis Access	264
Radial Artery Assessment	265
Rehab Unit Transfer Techniques	266
Restraints (Role of Nursing Assistant)	268
Seclusion Restraint (Behavioral Health)	269
Skin Burn, Care of	271
Skin Prep Using Tincture of Iodine	272
Staple/Clip Removal	273
Sterile Gloves, Applying	274
Sterile Technique	275
Subcutaneous Needle Placement	276
Tenckhoff Catheter	278
Tissue Therapy	280
Tracheal Suctioning	281
Tracheostomy Care	284
Tracheostomy Tube Dislodgement, Emergency Intervention	285
Transfer of Patient with Cervical Surgery and Patient with Shoulder Surgery	287
Transfer Patient with Lumbar Surgery	288
Transfer, Transport, Ambulation	290
Transportation of Postcatheterization Patients	291
Tuberculosis Skin Test	292
Urinary Catheterization	294
VAC: Negative Pressure Wound Therapy	295
Vacuum Assisted Closure Device (VACD) for Negative Pressure Wound Therapy (NPWT)	299
Venous Reflux Exam	304
Ventilator—Assessment of the Patient and Troubleshooting	305
Vital Signs (Observation Room)	307
Weights/Height	308
Wound Cultures	310
Wound Photography	312
Zoladex, Subcutaneous Injection of	313

MS—Medical-Surgical

Name: _____ Date: _____

Skill: Accessing Implantable Access Devices

Steps	Completed	Comments
1. Assembles equipment.		
2. Explains procedure to patient.		
3. Puts mask on self and patient.		
4. Prepares sterile field with equipment.		
5. Dons sterile gloves.		
6. Cleanses site with alcohol/povidone swab sticks per procedure.		
7. Palpates/locates portal septum and stabilizes.		
8. Inserts primed noncoring needle perpendicularly into center of septum; aspirates for blood return.		
9. With blood return injects N/S into port, clamps tubing and removes syringe.		
10. Flushes port according to procedure using positive pressure.		
11. Attaches primed prn adapter if indicated/initiates infusion.		
12. Applies dressing per procedure.		
13. Leaves capped tubing unclamped.		
14. Maintains strict sterile technique throughout procedure.		

Self-assessment	Evaluation/ validation methods	Levels	Type of validation	Comments
❏ Experienced ❏ Need practice ❏ Never done ❏ Not applicable (based on scope of practice)	❏ Verbal ❏ Demonstration/ observation ❏ Practical exercise ❏ Interactive class	❏ Beginner ❏ Intermediate ❏ Expert	❏ Orientation ❏ Annual ❏ Other _____	

_____ _____
Employee signature   *Observer signature*

Reference:
Duell, D., Martin, B., and Smith, S. 2008. *Clinical Nursing Skills: Basic to Advanced Skills.* 7th ed. Upper Saddle River, NJ: Pearson Education, Inc.

MS—Medical-Surgical

Name: _____ Date: _____

Skill: Adding IV Solution, Priming Tubing, Changing Tubing

Steps	Completed	Comments
1. Washes hands.		
2. Assembles equipment.		
3. Reviews physician's order.		
4. Chooses correct solution.		
5. Removes outer wrapper.		
6. Examines IV solution for clarity, particles; checks expiration date.		
7. Examines container for holes.		
8. Selects IV tubing appropriate to flow rate. Selects extension if indicated.		
9. Closes clamp(s) on IV.		
10. Inserts spike into IV port, holding neck of port.		
11. Squeezes drip chamber. Fills to appropriate level.		
12. Inverts IV bag and hangs on IV pole.		
13. Primes tubing.		
14. Explains procedure to patient.		
15. Dons gloves.		
16. Removes dressing if catheter/needle hub not visible.		
17. Places 2x2 under hub.		
18. Slows current IV solution.		
19. Disconnects old IV tubing while stabilizing hub with other hand.		
20. Connects new tubing while stabilizing hub.		
21. Initiates and regulates the infusion.		
22. Labels tubing and bag.		
23. Discards old tubing and gloves.		
24. Documents procedure including amount of fluid discharged.		

Evidence-Based Competency Management for the Medical-Surgical Unit, Second Edition

MS—Medical-Surgical

Self-assessment	Evaluation/ validation methods	Levels	Type of validation	Comments
❏ Experienced ❏ Need practice ❏ Never done ❏ Not applicable (based on scope of practice)	❏ Verbal ❏ Demonstration/ observation ❏ Practical exercise ❏ Interactive class	❏ Beginner ❏ Intermediate ❏ Expert	❏ Orientation ❏ Annual ❏ Other _____	

_____   _____
Employee signature   *Observer signature*

Reference:
Perry, A. and Potter, P. 2006. *Clinical Nursing Skills & Techniques.* 6th Ed. St. Louis, MO: Mosby Elsevier.

Name: _____ Date: _____

Skill: Adding IV Solution to Central Line

Steps	Completed	Comments
1. Washes hands.		
2. Assembles equipment.		
3. Reviews physician's orders.		
4. Chooses correct solution.		
5. Removes outer wrapper.		
6. Examines IV solution for clarity, particles; checks expiration date.		
7. Examines container for holes.		
8. Identifies proper IV line to add IV.		
9. Removes old IV bag from IV tubing.		
10. Inserts spike to IV port.		
11. Hangs new bag to IV pole.		
12. Programs correct volume to be infused on pump and begins to infuse.		
13. Documents new bag.		

Self-assessment	Evaluation/ validation methods	Levels	Type of validation	Comments
❏ Experienced ❏ Need practice ❏ Never done ❏ Not applicable (based on scope of practice)	❏ Verbal ❏ Demonstration/ observation ❏ Practical exercise ❏ Interactive class	❏ Beginner ❏ Intermediate ❏ Expert	❏ Orientation ❏ Annual ❏ Other _____	

_____ _____
Employee signature   *Observer signature*

Reference:
Perry, A. and Potter, P. 2006. *Clinical Nursing Skills & Techniques.* 6th Ed. St. Louis, MO: Mosby Elsevier.

MS—Medical-Surgical

Name: _____ Date: _____

Skill: Administration of Blood

Steps	Completed	Comments
1. Verifies the original physician's order and documentation of informed consent.		
2. Utilizes principles of body substance isolation, explains procedure to patient, and educates patient in symptoms to report to nurse.		
3. Obtains blood or blood component from the laboratory.		
a. The staff member calling for a unit of blood, must state both name and medical record number of the patient.		
b. Addressograph a blood component issue card and a red identification band. The person obtaining the blood/blood component and the blood bank technician verify that the name and medical record number on the issue card, the product chart copy, the red identification band, and the unit of blood are the same.		
4. Establishes IV at KO rate or per physician's order.		
a. Prime Y tubing with 250 cc normal saline solution.		
b. Follow procedure for starting IV It is recommended that an 18–20 gauge intravenous catheter/needle be used.		
5. Performs identification. A registered nurse and licensed practical nurse or licensed respiratory therapist or physician (one must be a registered nurse) must identify the patient receiving the blood/blood product by:		
a. Verifying the original physician's order and informed consent.		
b. Verifying the patient's name and ID number on the patient's name band matches the name and ID number on the compatibility tag on the blood/blood product, the product chart copy, and the red ID band.		

c. Verifying that the expiration date, the ABO/Rh compatibility, unit number printed on the blood/blood product label, and the product chart copy are the same and acceptable before the infusion. The persons who verify the blood product and identify the patient must sign the product copy chart.		
d. The red identification band is placed on the same extremity as the hospital identification band.		
6. Obtains vital signs: a. Pretransfusion vital signs are required, including a temperature. If vital signs have been taken within an hour, these may be used. b. The nurse remains with the patient for the first 15 minutes of the transfusion. c. Vital signs 15 minutes into the transfusion 30 minutes after that and then hourly until the infusion is complete. d. Monitors the patient every 30 minutes by looking for signs/symptoms of reaction/response to the transfusion. e. Posttransfusion vital signs are taken at the conclusion of the transfusion. The registered nurse responsible for the patient will monitor the vital signs and notify the physician when appropriate. This step may be delegated. However, the registered nurse responsible for the patient will monitor the assessment and notify the physician when appropriate.		
7. Attaches blood to tubing. Spikes the blood bag before hanging it up onto the pole. Checks filter and expresses air that might be trapped there before switching to blood.		
8. Upon completion of administration of blood, clears tubing with normal saline unless otherwise ordered and removes red ID band.		
9. Discontinues IV if ordered.		

MS—Medical-Surgical

10. Record patient's vital signs and reaction, if any, on product chart copy. If a transfusion reaction occurs, also complete the transfusion reaction investigation portion of the blood bank requisition form.		
11. Places product chart copy in the patient's medical chart.		
12. Disposes of blood bag and tubing in red plastic bag.		
13. Documents.		

Self-assessment	Evaluation/ validation methods	Levels	Type of validation	Comments
❏ Experienced ❏ Need practice ❏ Never done ❏ Not applicable (based on scope of practice)	❏ Verbal ❏ Demonstration/ observation ❏ Practical exercise ❏ Interactive class	❏ Beginner ❏ Intermediate ❏ Expert	❏ Orientation ❏ Annual ❏ Other _____	

Employee signature

Observer signature

Reference:
AABB. 2006. *Standards for blood bank and transfusions.* 24th ed. Bethesda, MD: AABB.

The Joint Commission. 2006. *Tubing misconnections – a persistent and potentially deadly occurrence.* www.jointcommission.org (retrieved May 25, 2006).

Perry, A. and Potter, P. 2006. *Fundamentals of Nursing.* 6th ed. St. Louis, MO: Mosby Elsevier.

Summa Health System. *Patient Care Services Policy and Procedure Manual: Care of the Suicidal/Homicidal Patient.*

MS—Medical-Surgical

Name: _____ Date: _____

Skill: **Applanation Tonometry**

Steps	Completed	Comments
1. Demonstrates proper process of identification of patient and eye to be tested.		
2. Demonstrates ability to explain procedure to patient.		
3. Demonstrates ability to instill the appropriate anesthetic eye drops to numb the eye being tested.		
4. Demonstrates proper setting of all appropriate dials on slit lamp.		
5. Demonstrates proper positioning of patient for procedure.		
6. Demonstrates ability to accurately measure and record IOP on medical record.		

Self-assessment	Evaluation/ validation methods	Levels	Type of validation	Comments
❏ Experienced ❏ Need practice ❏ Never done ❏ Not applicable (based on scope of practice)	❏ Verbal ❏ Demonstration/ observation ❏ Practical exercise ❏ Interactive class	❏ Beginner ❏ Intermediate ❏ Expert	❏ Orientation ❏ Annual ❏ Other _____	

_____   _____
Employee signature   ***Observer signature***

Reference:
American Ophthalmological Society. 2003. AOS Task Force on Curriculum in Ophthalmology for Medical Students.

MS—Medical-Surgical

Name: _____ Date: _____

Skill: **Appointment Scheduling—Clinic**

Steps	Completed	Comments
1. Determine accurate spelling of patient's full name and if patient has medical records number in Medipac.		
2. Establish correct visit type with appropriate information in note field.		
3. Explains in note field reason for overbooking of physician appointments.		
4. Documents patient insurance information.		
5. Verifies referral if necessary for visit.		
6. Documents in note field any test results patient will bring or if another agency is sending.		
7. If patient has not been a recent client, check to see if previous physician is still on staff. If not, assign as new patient to another practitioner.		

Self-assessment	Evaluation/ validation methods	Levels	Type of validation	Comments
❏ Experienced ❏ Need practice ❏ Never done ❏ Not applicable (based on scope of practice)	❏ Verbal ❏ Demonstration/ observation ❏ Practical exercise ❏ Interactive class	❏ Beginner ❏ Intermediate ❏ Expert	❏ Orientation ❏ Annual ❏ Other _____	

_____ _____
Employee signature   *Observer signature*

Reference:
Summa Health System. 2006. *Your Guide to Service Excellence.*

Name: _____ Date: _____

Skill: **Atrium Ocean (Wet) Chest Tube Collection Set-Up**

Steps	Completed	Comments
1. Verifies order, selects correct collection device, and opens plastic outer wrap.		
2. Removes blue wrapping, opens floor stand, and places unit upright on a flat surface.		
3. Fills water seal chamber to 2 cm line using Attached funnel.		
4. Fills suction control chamber.		

5. Connects drainage tube to chest tube.
If tube is newly inserted:
  a. Removes the patient tube connector cap and while keeping ends sterile, inserts securely into chest tube.
  b. Tapes the connection.		

6. **If changing collection unit of chest tube already in place:**
  a. Places new unit on floor near full unit.
  b. Removes drainage tube from new unit.
  c. Clamps drainage tube from patient and disconnects it from the full unit using padded hemostats.
  d. Attaches drainage tube to new unit.
  e. Releases hemostats.
  f. Reestablish suction if needed.		

7. **Applying suction**
  a. Obtains wall regulator and checks the filter.
  b. Inserts wall regulator into wall outlet.
  c. Connects suction source line directly to the suction control stopcock or suction connector on Atrium unit.
  d. Turn wall regulator to continuous suction with at least 80 mm suction and constant, gentle bubbling occurs in the suction control chamber.		

MS—Medical-Surgical

8. For Water Seal
  a. Leaves stopcock on top of unit in OPEN or ON position.
  b. Does not connect port to wall suction tubing.		

DOCUMENTATION **9. Interdisciplinary Clinical Pathway / Kardex:** a. Explanation of procedure to patient and significant others		
On Graphics / Intake and Output: a. Amount of drainage		

Interdisciplinary Progress Note:
  a. Change of chest tube collection chamber
  b. Presence / absence of air leak.		

Patient Progress Notes / Critical Care Flowsheet
  a. CT insertion to water seal/suction.
  b. Amount and color of initial drainage.
  c. Presence / absence of air leak.		

Self-assessment	Evaluation/ validation methods	Levels	Type of validation	Comments
❏ Experienced ❏ Need practice ❏ Never done ❏ Not applicable (based on scope of practice)	❏ Verbal ❏ Demonstration/ observation ❏ Practical exercise ❏ Interactive class	❏ Beginner ❏ Intermediate ❏ Expert	❏ Orientation ❏ Annual ❏ Other _____	

_____   _____
Employee signature   *Observer signature*

References:

Atrium Medical Corporation. 1993. *Managing Chest Drainage.* Hudson, NH: Atrium Medical Corporation.

Carlson, K. and Wiegand, D. 2005. AACN procedure manual for critical care. 5th ed. St. Louis, MO: Elsevier Mosby.

MS—Medical-Surgical

Name: _____ Date: _____

Skill: **Barthel Index—Modified Rankin Scale**

Steps	Completed	Comments
Critical Elements 1. Selects the appropriate score for the patient using the Barthel Index Scoring System (5, 10 or 15) for each area of activity:		
a. Feeding		
b. Bathing		
c. Grooming		
d. Dressing		
e. Bowel control		
f. Bladder control		
g. Toilet transfers		
h. Chair/bed transfers		
i. Ambulation		
j. Stairs		
2. Records performance in each category prior to admission and on admission by interviewing patient or family. If not already obtained.		
3. Enters Total Barthel Index Score and initials.		
4. Enters Modified Rankin Scale score as indicated by patients physical limitations into appropriate box.		
5. Enters initials as appropriate.		

Self-assessment	Evaluation/ validation methods	Levels	Type of validation	Comments

❏ Experienced
❏ Need practice
❏ Never done
❏ Not applicable
   (based on scope of
   practice)
	❏ Verbal
	❏ Demonstration/
	   observation
	❏ Practical exercise
	❏ Interactive class
		❏ Beginner
		❏ Intermediate
		❏ Expert
			❏ Orientation
			❏ Annual
			❏ Other _____	

_____ _____
Employee signature *Observer signature*

Reference:
Barthel, D., and Mahoney, F. 1965. Functional evaluation: the Barthel Index. *Maryland State Medical Journal* 14: 56-61.

Evidence-Based Competency Management for the Medical-Surgical Unit, Second Edition

MS—Medical-Surgical

Name: _____ Date: _____

Skill: Bed Bath

Steps	Completed	Comments
1. Utilizes principles of body substance isolation.		
2. Obtains all articles needed for hygiene and bed making.		
3. Removes top linen and place a bath blanket on patient, removes gown/pajamas.		
4. Offers urinal or bedpan. Empties container and washes own hands.		
5. Assists patient to the nearest side of the bed.		
6. Supplies equipment/assists with brushing the teeth and mouth care/cleans dentures.		
7. Washes face, ears, and neck. Rinses and dries.		
8. Washes, rinse, and dry arms, chest, abdomen, includes the area of the thighs near the groin.		
9. Applies deodorant under arms.		
10. Washes each leg and foot separately. Rinses and dries.		
11. Changes the water.		
12. Rolls the patient away from him or her. Places the towel along the back and turns the bath blanket back to expose the back and buttocks. Bends the upper leg (this keeps the patient in the side-lying position).		
13. Washes the back of the neck, the back, the buttocks, and the upper thighs. Rinses and dries. (Do not wash the rectal area at this time.)		
14. Rubs the patient's back with lotion.		
15. Washes the pubic area (or patient washes this area, if able).		
16. Turns patient on side again, washes, rinses, and dries the rectal area.		
17. Protects the bed with the towel and combs the back of the hair.		
18. Turns onto back and finishes combing the hair.		
19. Supplies clean gown/pajamas.		
20. Makes bed.		

Self-assessment	Evaluation/ validation methods	Levels	Type of validation	Comments
❏ Experienced ❏ Need practice ❏ Never done ❏ Not applicable (based on scope of practice)	❏ Verbal ❏ Demonstration/ observation ❏ Practical exercise ❏ Interactive class	❏ Beginner ❏ Intermediate ❏ Expert	❏ Orientation ❏ Annual ❏ Other _____	

Employee signature *Observer signature*

Reference:
Alvare, S., Dugan, D., and Fuzy, J. 2005. *Nursing Assistant Care*. Albuquerque, NM: Hartman Publishing.

MS—Medical-Surgical

Name: _____ Date: _____

Skill: **BICAP and Cautery**

Steps	Completed	Comments
1. Names and locates all cautery setups in the endoscopy department.		
2. Demonstrates correct way to set up the Microvasive ENDOSTAT II on emergency cart. a. Bicap – Correct set-up		
b. Cautery – Correct set-up		
3. Demonstrates the correct way to connect the gold probe on the emergency cart and on the regular Bicap. a. Gold Probe — regular		
b. Gold Probe with needle		
4. Explain the difference between a monopolar and bipolar cautery.		
5. Demonstrates the set-up of a valley lab unit.		
6. Demonstrate the set-up of a Surgistat unit.		
7. Demonstrate proper grounding pad placement.		
8. Demonstrate the proper set-up of the E.R.C.P. cautery unit (Valley Lab). a. Proper settings		
b. Correct cautery cords for each papillatome used. 1. Wilson cook		
2. Microvasive		
3. Bard		

Self-assessment	Evaluation/ validation methods	Levels	Type of validation	Comments
❏ Experienced ❏ Need practice ❏ Never done ❏ Not applicable (based on scope of practice)	❏ Verbal ❏ Demonstration/ observation ❏ Practical exercise ❏ Interactive class	❏ Beginner ❏ Intermediate ❏ Expert	❏ Orientation ❏ Annual ❏ Other _____	

_____   _____
Employee signature   *Observer signature*

Reference:
American Society for Gastrointestinal Endoscopy. 2002. Complications of upper GI endoscopy. *Gastrointestinal Endoscopy* 55(7): 784-793.

MS—Medical-Surgical

Name: _____ Date: _____

Skill: Bladder Scan

Steps	Completed	Comments
1. Place patient in supine position; expose abdomen to symphysis pubis.		
2. Press on button, press scan button.		
3. Select gender. **NOTE: When the woman has had a hysterectomy, the gender is set as male.**		
4. Apply ultrasound gel to the dome of the probe and 1-2 inches above the symphysis pubis, mid line. **NOTE: Remove air bubbles from the gel as this may block transmission.**		
5. Make sure the head on the patient icon of the probe points to the patient's head when the probe is placed on abdomen.		
6. Once placed on abdomen, angle probe slightly downward. Press and release the scan button.		
7. Press done for Scan Results screen. Press print button twice to print results. Document in interdisciplinary progress note: Date, time, amount, time since last void, notification of physician.		
8. Wipe off gel from abdomen and re-cover area. Wipe off probe with dry paper towel. **NOTE: Do not use water.**		

Self-assessment	Evaluation/ validation methods	Levels	Type of validation	Comments
❏ Experienced ❏ Need practice ❏ Never done ❏ Not applicable (based on scope of practice)	❏ Verbal ❏ Demonstration/ observation ❏ Practical exercise ❏ Interactive class	❏ Beginner ❏ Intermediate ❏ Expert	❏ Orientation ❏ Annual ❏ Other _____	

_____ _____
Employee signature   *Observer signature*

Reference:
Diagnostic Ultrasound. 2001. *Urology for Primary Care.*

Byun, S., et al. 2003. Three dimension ultrasound bladder scanner predicts bladder volumes with good accuracy. *Urology* 62: 656-660.

Evidence-Based Competency Management for the Medical-Surgical Unit, Second Edition

MS—Medical-Surgical

Name: _____ Date: _____

Skill: **Blood Culture Collection**

Steps	Completed	Comments
1. Obtains equipment (requisition, labels, aerobic/anaerobic bottles, alcohol swabs, Frepp chorhexidine prep, sterile 20 mL syringes, and sterile needles).		
2. Identifies and describes procedure to patient.		
3. Applies tourniquet to patient's arm, locates venipuncture site, and removes tourniquet.		
4. Prepares venipuncture site: • Applies Frepp chlorhexidine to site of entry using side-to-side friction for 30 seconds Allows to air dry for 30 seconds.		
5. Disinfects rubber tops of each bottle with alcohol. Allows to air dry.		
6. Assembles need and syringe.		
7. Reapplies tourniquet above venipuncture site taking care to avoid site contamination. Does not repalpate site.		
8. Dons gloves.		
9. With bevel side up, introduces needle into vein and slowly draws plunger back until volume in syringe reaches 20 mL.		
10. Removes needle and applies cotton ball with pressure to site.		
11. Inserts needle into aerobic bottle first and dispenses 8–10 mL of blood.		
12. Removes syringe/needle from aerobic bottle and inserts into anaerobic bottle dispensing 8–10 mL of blood.		
13. Identifies the following criteria: • Each bottle must have a minimum of 5 mL of blood • If less than 10 mL is collected, then 5 mL is put into the aerobic bottle and the remainder into the anaerobic bottle		

MS—Medical-Surgical

14. Labels each bottle (patient name, room number, medical record number, time/date drawn, and initials of person drawing). Also notes number of culture set (#1, #2, etc.). Does not cover bar code with label.		
15. Marks date/time drawn and initials/signature with employee identification number on requisition.		
16. Inverts each bottle three or four times to mix blood, media, and anticoagulant.		
17. Sends specimens to microbiology.		
18. Documents procedure and patient tolerance.		

Self-assessment	Evaluation/ validation methods	Levels	Type of validation	Comments
❏ Experienced ❏ Need practice ❏ Never done ❏ Not applicable (based on scope of practice)	❏ Verbal ❏ Demonstration/ observation ❏ Practical exercise ❏ Interactive class	❏ Beginner ❏ Intermediate ❏ Expert	❏ Orientation ❏ Annual ❏ Other _____	

_____   _____
Employee signature   **Observer signature**

Reference:
Springhouse Corporation. 2004. *Nursing Procedures*. 4th ed. Philadelphia, PA: Lippincott Williams & Wilkin.

MS—Medical-Surgical

Name: _____ Date: _____

Skill: Braden Scale

Steps	Completed	Comments
1. Selects appropriate score for the following categories using Braden Scale definitions: 　a. sensory perceptions		
b. Moisture		
c. Activity		
d. Mobility		
e. Nutrition		
f. Function and shear		
2. Records score in each category upon admission.		
3. Enters total score.		
4. Identifies when to notify wound care center.		
5. Identifies daily reassessment of moderate-high-risk patients and every three-day assessment of low-risk patients.		

Self-assessment	Evaluation/ validation methods	Levels	Type of validation	Comments
❑ Experienced ❑ Need practice ❑ Never done ❑ Not applicable (based on scope of practice)	❑ Verbal ❑ Demonstration/ observation ❑ Practical exercise ❑ Interactive class	❑ Beginner ❑ Intermediate ❑ Expert	❑ Orientation ❑ Annual ❑ Other _____	

_____ _____
Employee signature　　　　　　　　　　　　*Observer signature*

Reference:
Perry, A. and Potter, P. 2006. *Clinical Nursing Skills & Techniques.* 6th ed. St. Louis, MO: Mosby Elsevier.

Name: _____ Date: _____

Skill: CADD Pump

Steps	Completed	Comments
I. Pump set-up: 1. Inserts alkaline battery.		
2. Attaches medication cassette.		
3. Connects tubing.		
4. Ensures tubing is primed and air-free.		
5. Reviews order sheet.		
II. Pump programming: 1. Stops pump.		
2. Places pump in LLO.		
3. Programs residual volume.		
4. Programs medication concentration.		
5. Programs continuous infusion rate.		
6. Programs PCA dose.		
7. Sets lock-out time (doses/hr. and doses/min.).		
8. Clears dose given screen.		
9. Clears total dose given screen.		
10. Places pump in LL2.		
11. Restarts pump.		
III. Bag changing: 1. Stops pump.		
2. Places pump in LLO.		
3. Attaches bag.		
4. Programs residual volume.		
5. Place pump in LL2.		
6. Documents bag change.		
IV. Documentation: 1. Documents on progress record:		
A. Time		
B. Medication		
C. Dose		
D. Rate/hour		
E. Pain scale		
F. Site		

Evidence-Based Competency Management for the Medical-Surgical Unit, Second Edition

MS—Medical-Surgical

2. Documents the following guidelines on pain control flow sheet once per shift:		
A. Time		
B. Dose given		
C. Basal infusion		
D. Respiratory rate		
E. Pain scale		
F. Nausea and vomiting		
G. Purities		
H. Urinary retention		
I. Sensory level		

Self-assessment	Evaluation/ validation methods	Levels	Type of validation	Comments
❑ Experienced ❑ Need practice ❑ Never done ❑ Not applicable (based on scope of practice)	❑ Verbal ❑ Demonstration/ observation ❑ Practical exercise ❑ Interactive class	❑ Beginner ❑ Intermediate ❑ Expert	❑ Orientation ❑ Annual ❑ Other _____	

_____   _____
Employee signature   ***Observer signature***

Reference:
September–October 2001. Patient-controlled analgesic infusion pumps: Evaluating the Deltec CADD-Prizm PCS II. *Health Devices* 30(9-10): 360-364.

MS—Medical-Surgical

Name: _____   Date: _____

Skill: Care of the Patient with Central Venous Catheters

Steps	Completed	Comments
A. General Care of Central Venous Catheters		
1. States prescribed days to change IV tubings and dressings and stopcock.		
2. States prescribed day to change infusion plugs.		
3. Documents.		
B. Placing and Using Clave Adapters		
1. Gathers supplies.		
2. Places patient in a supine position unless contraindicated.		
3. Sanitize hands.		
4. Clamps, tails using <u>padded</u> hemostat or the provided slide clamp before removing the existing infusion plug or IV tubing.		
5. With tails clamped removes previous injection cap, removes the plastic end from the new sterile injection cap and connects primed plug to the hub of the lumen or catheter.		
6. Cleans the injection cap with alcohol for 30."		
7. Remove previous adapter. Cleanse catheter hub with alcohol wipe being careful <u>not</u> to wipe over "open end" of pigtail hub.		
8. Apply sterile, primed Clave adapter.		
9. Using friction, cleanse Clave adapter with alcohol wipe.		
10. Dispose of soiled supplies, remove gloves, and perform hand hygiene.		
11. Discuss SAS method of flush.		
12. Documents.		

Evidence-Based Competency Management for the Medical-Surgical Unit, Second Edition

MS—Medical-Surgical

Self-assessment	Evaluation/ validation methods	Levels	Type of validation	Comments
❏ Experienced ❏ Need practice ❏ Never done ❏ Not applicable (based on scope of practice)	❏ Verbal ❏ Demonstration/ observation ❏ Practical exercise ❏ Interactive class	❏ Beginner ❏ Intermediate ❏ Expert	❏ Orientation ❏ Annual ❏ Other _____	

_____

Employee signature

_____

Observer signature

Reference:
Weinstein, S. 2007. *Plumer's Principles and Practice of Intravenous Therapy.* 8th ed. Philadelphia, PA: Lippincott.

Name: _____ Date: _____

Skill: Central Venous Catheter—Application of Sterile Occlusive Dressing

Steps	Completed	Comments
1. Obtains central venous catheter dressing kit and other necessary supplies.		
2. Turns off nearby fans, covers air vents near patient bed, pulls curtains around bed, closes door.		
3. Explains procedure to patient. Places patient in a supine position with head turned away from catheter site, unless contraindicated.		
4. Washes hands, dons mask, applies clean gloves.		
5. Removes dressing. Clips hair as necessary.		
6. Removes gloves; applies second sterile pair.		
7. Cleans catheter insertion site with gauze soaked in normal saline.		
8. Inspects site. Notes condition of exposed catheter.		
9. Cleans catheter site with povidone iodine swabsticks.		
10. Applies povidone iodine ointment to insertion site and sutures sites.		
11. Places slit gauze on top of insertion site.		
12. Places a second piece of gauze.		
13. Applies skin adherent preparation/tape.		
14. Applies strips of overlapping tape or transparent dressing. Uses a half-split piece of tape under pigtails.		
15. Changes IV tubing.		
16. Labels dressing with date of insertion, date of dressing change, and initials.		
17. Loops tubing over dressing and secure with tape.		
18. Document on patient progress record and Kardex.		

MS—Medical-Surgical

Self-assessment	Evaluation/ validation methods	Levels	Type of validation	Comments
❏ Experienced ❏ Need practice ❏ Never done ❏ Not applicable (based on scope of practice)	❏ Verbal ❏ Demonstration/ observation ❏ Practical exercise ❏ Interactive class	❏ Beginner ❏ Intermediate ❏ Expert	❏ Orientation ❏ Annual ❏ Other _____	

_____   _____
Employee signature   ***Observer signature***

Reference:
Perry, A. and Potter, P. 2006. *Clinical Nursing Skills & Techniques.* 6th ed. St. Louis, MO: Mosby Elsevier.

MS—Medical-Surgical

Name: _____ Date: _____

Skill: **Central Venous Catheter—Obtaining Blood Samples**

Steps	Completed	Comments
I. Placing and using three-way stopcock for blood draws.		
1. Gathers equipment.		
2. Stops all infusion. Explains procedure to patient and places patient supine, unless contraindicated.		
3. Washes hands. Puts on gloves.		
4. Stops IV infusions through all lumens of central line (including introducer) 30 seconds prior to and while drawing blood samples.		
5. Clamps proximal pigtail.		
6. Cleanses catheter hub/tubing connection with alcohol wipe.		
7. Maintaining aseptic technique, attaches IV line to stopcock, and flushes IV fluid.		
8. Cleanses catheter hub with alcohol wipe using friction. Attaches stopcock to catheter.		
9. Places primed Clave adapter on stopcock side-port. Unclamps proximal pigtail.		
10. Turns stopcock off to the IV fluid and open to Clave adapter. Cleanses Clave adapter stopcock with alcohol wipe, using friction.		
11. Attaches 10-cc syringe filled with 5 mL of normal saline and flush.		
12. Inserts vacutainer sleeve into Clave adapter. Discards 5 mL blood sample.		
13. Draws blood samples using appropriate tubes.		
14. Turns stopcock off to Clave adapter.		
15. Removes vacutainer sleeve from PRN adapter.		
16. Attaches 10-mL or larger syringe containing 10 mL normal saline; opens stopcock to Clave adapter; flushes Clave or flushes stopcock with IV solution.		
17. Turns stopcock off to Clave adapter and opens to IV fluid. Restarts infusion(s) ordered.		

Evidence-Based Competency Management for the Medical-Surgical Unit, Second Edition

MS—Medical-Surgical

18. Sends labeled blood to lab.			
19. Marks lab requisition that blood was drawn from a central line.			
II. Obtaining blood samples through clave adapter			
1. Stops IV infusions through all lumens 30 seconds prior to and while drawing blood samples.			
2. Places patient supine position unless contraindicated.			
3. Thoroughly cleanses Clave adapter with alcohol swab using friction.			
4. Inserts 10-cc syringe filled with 5 mL or normal saline flush using a pushing twisting method and flush line.			
5. Inserts vacutainer sleeve into Clave adapter. Discards a 5-mL blood sample. Inserts appropriate tubes to draw desired blood samples.			
6. Removes vacutainer sleeve from Clave adapter.			
7. Flushes with 10-mL normal saline using a pushing twisting motion to connect syringe.			
8. Sends labeled blood to lab and writes on requisition that blood was drawn from a central line.			
9. Restarts infusion(s), if applicable.			

Self-assessment	Evaluation/ validation methods	Levels	Type of validation	Comments
❏ Experienced ❏ Need practice ❏ Never done ❏ Not applicable (based on scope of practice)	❏ Verbal ❏ Demonstration/ observation ❏ Practical exercise ❏ Interactive class	❏ Beginner ❏ Intermediate ❏ Expert	❏ Orientation ❏ Annual ❏ Other _____	

_____   _____
Employee signature   *Observer signature*

Reference:
Weinstein, S. 2007. *Plumer's Principles and Practice of Intravenous Therapy*. 8th ed. Philadelphia, PA: Lippincott.

Name: _____ Date: _____

Skill: Central Venous Catheter—Removal

Steps	Completed	Comments
1. Verify length of catheter.		
2. Explain procedure to patient.		
3. Apply mask.		
4. Prepare sterile field and assemble supplies: • Central line dressing kit • Sterile suture set (two if culture needed) • Sterile container for catheter tip		
5. Turn off IV solution to catheter.		
6. Place patient flat or in Trendelenburg as tolerated.		
7. Apply clean gloves.		
8. Remove tape and dressing.		
9. Apply sterile gloves.		
10. Cleanse catheter insertion site with Chloraprep swab in circular/outward motion. Allow to dry.		
11. Remove sutures.		
12. Instruct patient to exhale, hold breath, and bear down (if possible).		
13. Withdraw catheter slowly.		
14. Apply gauze to site and apply pressure for five minutes.		
15. Apply occlusive transparent dressing.		
16. Observe catheter tip for rough edges.		
17. If ordered, send catheter tip to Microbiology Department after placing in sterile culture tube.		
18. Patient to remain flat postprocedure. Assess patient for respiratory distress or bleeding.		
19. Document date and time of catheter removal, description site, integrity of catheter, and patient tolerance.		

MS—Medical-Surgical

Self-assessment	Evaluation/ validation methods	Levels	Type of validation	Comments
❏ Experienced ❏ Need practice ❏ Never done ❏ Not applicable (based on scope of practice)	❏ Verbal ❏ Demonstration/ observation ❏ Practical exercise ❏ Interactive class	❏ Beginner ❏ Intermediate ❏ Expert	❏ Orientation ❏ Annual ❏ Other _____	

_____   _____
Employee signature   *Observer signature*

Reference:
Weinstein, S. 2007. *Plumer's Principles and Practice of Intravenous Therapy*. 8th ed. Philadelphia, PA: Lippincott.

MS—Medical-Surgical

Name: _____   Date: _____

Skill: **Chemotherapy Administration**

Steps	Completed	Comments
1. Checks appropriate laboratory date prior to administering chemotherapy.		
2. Verifies physician's written order for specific dosage, route, cycle #, and mode of administration.		
3. Calculates drug dosage based on patient's height and weight and verifies dose is correct for cancer type.		
4. Clarifies any discrepancy with pharmacist/physician.		
5. Observes precautions in drug preparation and handling.		
6. Correctly states all potential side effects of the drugs.		
7. Checks all parameters of dispensed chemotherapy against the entire order with a second licensed person (RN, physician, pharmacist).		
8. Uses proper procedure to identify patient.		
9. Completes chemotherapy administration checklist.		
10. Assures patient comfort; provides antiemetic if indicated.		
11. Explains procedure and any side effects of the drugs. Answers patient's questions appropriately.		
12. Assesses patient's response to previous therapy.		
13. Teaches patient to report any adverse reactions immediately.		
14. Successfully performs venipuncture with two (or fewer) attempts.		
15. Checks patency of vein by instilling 5–7 cc of normal saline.		
16. Periodically reconfirms vein patency by obtaining blood backflow.		

Evidence-Based Competency Management for the Medical-Surgical Unit, Second Edition

MS—Medical-Surgical

17. Flushes tubing upon completion of one drug before administering another drug.		
18. Injects drugs at the appropriate speed to prevent untoward sensations/complications.		
19. Takes appropriate actions should infiltration of a drug occur.		
20. Observes for allergic or hypersensitivity reactions to the drugs and takes appropriate action should either occur.		
21. If using a venous access device, demonstrates skill in usage and maintenance of the device.		
22. Flushes intravenous tubing with a sufficient amount of saline to clear the line prior to removing the needle.		
23. Instructs patient on posttreatment care and precautions.		
24. Disposes of equipment in proper container.		
25. Documents procedure in the medical record.		

Self-assessment	Evaluation/ validation methods	Levels	Type of validation	Comments
❑ Experienced ❑ Need practice ❑ Never done ❑ Not applicable (based on scope of practice)	❑ Verbal ❑ Demonstration/ observation ❑ Practical exercise ❑ Interactive class	❑ Beginner ❑ Intermediate ❑ Expert	❑ Orientation ❑ Annual ❑ Other _____	

_____   _____
Employee signature   *Observer signature*

Reference:
Oncology Nursing Society. 2005. *Chemotherapy and Biotherapy Guidelines and Recommendations for Practice.* 2nd ed. Pennsylvania: Oncology Nursing Society (ONS).

MS—Medical-Surgical

Name: _____ Date: _____

Skill: Chemotherapy Teaching

Steps	Completed	Comments
1. Assesses patient's learning needs.		
a. What does patient already know about chemotherapy?		
b. What does patient want to know about chemotherapy?		
c. What is important for the patient to know about his or her chemotherapy?		
d. Does the patient have any cultural or religious barriers to learning?		
e. Is the patient ready, willing, and able to learn? • Physical limitations • Cognitive limitations		
f. Can the patient read, write, and understand English?		
g. Are there financial implications that will affect the patient's learning?		
2. Plans the education that is needed.		
3. Gives the appropriate handouts and educates the patient and family:		
A. Name of the medication		
B. Classification of medication		
C. Treatment regimen		
D. Expected side effects		
E. How to combat side effects		
F. Symptoms to call the doctor with		
G. Who/how to call the doctor		
4. Evaluates patient and family learning.		
5. Documents education and patient and family's response to education.		
6. Documents procedure in the medical record.		

Evidence-Based Competency Management for the Medical-Surgical Unit, Second Edition

MS—Medical-Surgical

Self-assessment	Evaluation/ validation methods	Levels	Type of validation	Comments
❑ Experienced ❑ Need practice ❑ Never done ❑ Not applicable (based on scope of practice)	❑ Verbal ❑ Demonstration/ observation ❑ Practical exercise ❑ Interactive class	❑ Beginner ❑ Intermediate ❑ Expert	❑ Orientation ❑ Annual ❑ Other _____	

_____   _____
Employee signature   *Observer signature*

Reference:
Duell, D., Martin, B., and Smith, S. 2008. *Clinical Nursing Skills: Basic to Advanced Skills*. 7th ed. Upper Saddle River, NJ: Pearson Education, Inc.

MS—Medical-Surgical

Name: _____ Date: _____

Skill: Chest Drainage Autotransfusion—Atrium Unit

Steps	Completed	Comments
A. **Autotransfusion — Blood recovery** * This procedure must be completed within four hours of chest/mediastinal tube insertion. 1. Verbalizes this procedure must be completed within four hours of chest/mediastinal tube insertion.		
2. Gathers equipment and takes to bedside Atrium ATS Bag, Pall Filter, blood tubing, and bag of 0.9% NS.		
3. Closes the chest drain ATS (autotransfusion) access line clamp and the ATS bag clamp.		
4. Removes the spike port cap and inserts the ATS bag spike into the chest drain ATS access line spike port using a firm twisting motion.		
5. Holds the ATS bag below the chest drain and opens both clamps.		
6. Gently bends the ATS bag upward where indicated to activate blood transfer. a. If ATS bag is accidentally activated prior to system connection, simply displace air into the Chest Drain after system connection.		
7. Once blood evacuation is completed, closes both clamps (ATS access line and ATS blood bag) and removes the ATS access line spike from the ATS access line spike port with a firm twisting motion.		
8. Inserts the ATS access line spike into the ATS bag spike holder.		
9. Recaps the access line using sterile technique and repositions the tubing in its holder.		
B. **Autotransfusion — Reinfusion** 1. Primes nonvented IV blood administration tubing and microembolic filter with normal saline.		

MS—Medical-Surgical

2. Attaches filter first to y-tubing and allows NS to penetrate/moistens filter.		
3. Removes ATS bag cap and attaches to filter spike.		
4. Connects the ATS bag, opens the clamp, and administers the autotransfusion. a. A pressure bag can be placed over the ATS bag to increase the flow rate if needed		
5. Documents the procedure. a. In progress record — Autotransfusion and amount b. On I&O — Autotransfusion — Amount		

Self-assessment	Evaluation/ validation methods	Levels	Type of validation	Comments
❏ Experienced ❏ Need practice ❏ Never done ❏ Not applicable (based on scope of practice)	❏ Verbal ❏ Demonstration/ observation ❏ Practical exercise ❏ Interactive class	❏ Beginner ❏ Intermediate ❏ Expert	❏ Orientation ❏ Annual ❏ Other _____	

_____   _____
Employee signature   *Observer signature*

Reference:
Kala, T., Matsuno, Y., Sekino, S., Takagi, H., and Umemoto, T. 2007. Intraoperative autotransfusion in abdominal aortic aneurysm surgery: Meta-analysis of randomized controlled trials. *Archives of Surgery* 142(11): 1098-1101.

MS—Medical-Surgical

Name: _____ Date: _____

Skill: **Chest Tube Dressing Change**

Steps	Completed	Comments
1. Verifies physician preference for petroleum gauze strip/antibiotic ointment around and next to skin. If not specified, uses only vaseline gauze.		
2. Gathers equipment and takes to bedside.		
3. Prepares sterile field with dressing change supplies.		
4. Wearing clean gloves, removes dressing, and discards.		
5. With sterile glove, cleanses site with 3x4 gauze and sterile normal saline.		
6. Observes markings on chest tube (centimeters chest tube is inserted).		
7. Applies antibiotic ointment to site with sterile applicator, if ordered.		
8. Wraps vaseline gauze strip around tube and over site.		
9. Places fenestrated (split) dressing around tube.		
10. Places sterile 4x3 gauze pads over insertion site (top and bottom) with tube exiting in center.		
11. Tears strips of two-inch tape, secures dressing by overlapping each piece of tape, shingling to achieve an occlusive dressing.		
12. Labels dressing with date, time, and initials.		
13. Documents, including first centimeter mark exposed at insertion site and centimeter mark that is exposed outside of dressing.		

Self-assessment	Evaluation/ validation methods	Levels	Type of validation	Comments
❏ Experienced ❏ Need practice ❏ Never done ❏ Not applicable (based on scope of practice)	❏ Verbal ❏ Demonstration/ observation ❏ Practical exercise ❏ Interactive class	❏ Beginner ❏ Intermediate ❏ Expert	❏ Orientation ❏ Annual ❏ Other _____	

_____ _____
Employee signature   *Observer signature*

Reference:
Perry, A. and Potter, P. 2006. *Clinical Nursing Skills & Techniques.* 6th ed. St. Louis, MO: Mosby Elsevier.

MS—Medical-Surgical

Name: _____ Date: _____

Skill: Code Management/Med-Surg

Steps	Completed	Comments
1. Assesses responsiveness		

2. If no response, calls for help from others on unit
   a. If unable to find someone, make stat call using phone in room
   b. Verbalizes correct phone number for Summa's Stat Line
		Asks for cart and AED
		
		(757)

3. Assesses breathing a. Opens airway		Look, Listen, Feel > 5 < 10 sec Head tilt/chin lift or jaw thrust

4. If patient is breathing:
   - Apply O2 via NC
   - Place heart monitor on patient
   - Place pulse oximeter on patient
   - Contact physician		

5. If patient is not breathing opens airway and provides 2 ventilations using mouth-to-mask, other barrier device, or ambu bag.		Make sure the chest rises.
6. Assesses pulse.		Checks >5 <10 sec

7. If no pulse begins chest compressions
   a. Verbalizes compression: ventilation ratio
   b. Compressions are 1 ½ - 2" deep
   c. Allows for complete chest recoil
   d. Compression rate is at least 100/min.
		30:2
		
		Compressions and ventilations continue until AED advises to clear patient.

8. When cart and second rescuer arrive
   a. Places back board under patient
   b. Turns on AED and follows prompts		

9. If "no shock advised" per AED, continues compressions/ventilations till Code Team arrives.		

10. Assigns roles as indicated
   a. When additional help arrives.
     1. Set up suction
     2. Assure/start patent peripheral IV
     3. Get patient's chart to bedside
     4. Be prepared to provide Code Team with brief history of events
		May elect to take one of these roles but should not leave patient's room.

MS—Medical-Surgical

11. Completes the top portion of the Team Record: date, unit, time team called, time team arrived, time CPR began, time AED placed, time defibrillated via AED.		
12. Participates in review of Code.		

Self-assessment	Evaluation/ validation methods	Levels	Type of validation	Comments
❏ Experienced ❏ Need practice ❏ Never done ❏ Not applicable (based on scope of practice)	❏ Verbal ❏ Demonstration/ observation ❏ Practical exercise ❏ Interactive class	❏ Beginner ❏ Intermediate ❏ Expert	❏ Orientation ❏ Annual ❏ Other _____	

_____   _____

Employee signature   ***Observer signature***

Reference:
American Heart Association. 2005. *BLS for Healthcare Providers.* Dallas, TX: AHA.

MS—Medical-Surgical

Name: _____ Date: _____

Skill: Conscious Sedation

Steps	Completed	Comments
1. Reviews the conscious sedation policy.		
2. Reviews/obtains patient history prior to procedure.		
3. Assesses for conditions compromising the airway, allergies, and general health status.		
4. Utilizes monitoring devices:		
• Cardiac monitoring		
• Blood pressure		
• Pulse oximetry		
5. Ascertains patency of IV access.		
6. Verifies availability of emergency equipment:		
• Suction		
• Oxygen		
• Reversal agents		
• Recognizes location of emergency cart and defibrillator for quick access		
7. Administers conscious sedation agent safely according to policy/rolodex guidelines.		
8. Records vital signs every 5 minutes during procedure.		
9. Remains with patient at all times and provides constant observation until recovered.		
10. Monitors signs & symptoms of respiratory depression.		
11. Monitors patient's ability to control secretions, swallow and cough.		
12. Takes vital signs q 15 minutes or more often as required postprocedure until v/s are consistent with baseline, no signs of respiratory distress and easily arousable to verbal stimuli.		
13. Documents procedure and patient outcome.		

MS—Medical-Surgical

Self-assessment	Evaluation/ validation methods	Levels	Type of validation	Comments
❏ Experienced ❏ Need practice ❏ Never done ❏ Not applicable (based on scope of practice)	❏ Verbal ❏ Demonstration/ observation ❏ Practical exercise ❏ Interactive class	❏ Beginner ❏ Intermediate ❏ Expert	❏ Orientation ❏ Annual ❏ Other _____	

_____   _____
Employee signature   *Observer signature*

Reference:
Bryan, R. 1997. Administering conscious sedation: Operational guidelines. *Critical Care Nursing Clinics of North America* 9(3): 289-300.

MS—Medical-Surgical

Name: _____ Date: _____

Skill: Conversion to Intermittent Infusion of Continuous IV

Steps	Completed	Comments
1. Assembles equipment:		
a. Intermittent infusion cap/J loop		
b. Alcohol swabs		
c. Normal saline (NS)		
d. 2x2		
e. Tape		
f. 2–3 cc needless syringe		
g. Gloves.		
2. Explains procedure.		
3. Prepares equipment.		
4. Washes hands.		
5. Cleanses NS vial, draws up 2 cc of NS.		
6. Primes injection cap & J loop with NS.		
7. Dons gloves.		
8. Places 2x2 under hub of needle.		
9. Clamps and disconnects IV tubing.		
10. Attaches intermittent injection cap with "J" loop.		
11. Cleanses cap. Inserts needle/syringe and verifies blood return, injects NS.		
12. Removes NS syringes.		
13. Tapes intermittent site.		
14. Removes gloves.		
15. Documents procedure and observation.		

Self-assessment	Evaluation/ validation methods	Levels	Type of validation	Comments
❏ Experienced ❏ Need practice ❏ Never done ❏ Not applicable (based on scope of practice)	❏ Verbal ❏ Demonstration/ observation ❏ Practical exercise ❏ Interactive class	❏ Beginner ❏ Intermediate ❏ Expert	❏ Orientation ❏ Annual ❏ Other _____	

_____

Employee signature

_____

Observer signature

Reference:
Perry, A. and Potter, P. 2006. *Clinical Nursing Skills & Techniques.* 6th ed. St. Louis, MO: Mosby Elsevier.

MS—Medical-Surgical

Name: _____ Date: _____

Skill: Crutch Walking and Use of Walker

Steps	Completed	Comments
Crutches:		
1. Demonstrates fitting crutches for a patient.		
2. Demonstrates crutch walking on level surface.		
3. Demonstrates procedure for staircase maneuvers: a. Going upstairs b. Going downstairs		
4. Demonstrate getting in and out of chair while using crutches.		
Walkers:		
1. Demonstrates fitting walker for a patient.		
2. Demonstrates using walker on level surface.		
3. Demonstrates using walker with steps: a. Going upstairs b. Going downstairs		

Self-assessment	Evaluation/ validation methods	Levels	Type of validation	Comments
❑ Experienced ❑ Need practice ❑ Never done ❑ Not applicable (based on scope of practice)	❑ Verbal ❑ Demonstration/ observation ❑ Practical exercise ❑ Interactive class	❑ Beginner ❑ Intermediate ❑ Expert	❑ Orientation ❑ Annual ❑ Other _____	

_____   _____

Employee signature   *Observer signature*

Reference:
Perry, A. and Potter, P. 2006. *Clinical Nursing Skills & Techniques.* 6th ed. St. Louis, MO: Mosby Elsevier.

MS—Medical-Surgical

Name: _____   Date: _____

Skill: Discontinuing IV Therapy

Steps	Completed	Comments
1. States reason for discontinuance.		
a. Order		
b. Infiltration		
c. Inflammation		
d. Increased pt c/o		
2. Assembles equipment.		
a. Sterile 4x3		
b. Bandage		
3. Washes hands. Applies gloves.		
4. Explains procedure to patient.		
5. Stops infusion, opens 4x3.		
6. Loosens tape. Removes dressing.		
7. Removes tape at site.		
8. Applies 4x3 at site with nondominant hand.		
9. Withdraws catheter or needle by pulling back from puncture site.		
10. States length of time to apply pressure.		
11. Assesses site.		
12. Applies bandage, if needed.		
13. Disposes of equipment. Maintains BSI.		
14. Documents procedure and observation findings.		

Self-assessment	Evaluation/ validation methods	Levels	Type of validation	Comments
❏ Experienced ❏ Need practice ❏ Never done ❏ Not applicable (based on scope of practice)	❏ Verbal ❏ Demonstration/ observation ❏ Practical exercise ❏ Interactive class	❏ Beginner ❏ Intermediate ❏ Expert	❏ Orientation ❏ Annual ❏ Other _____	

_____   _____
Employee signature   *Observer signature*

Reference:
Weinstein, S. 2007. *Plumer's Principles and Practice of Intravenous Therapy.* 8th ed. Philadelphia, PA: Lippincott.

Evidence-Based Competency Management for the Medical-Surgical Unit, Second Edition

MS—Medical-Surgical

Name: _____ Date: _____

Skill: Drug Testing, Blood and Urine

Steps	Completed	Comments
1. Identifies company requesting test.		
2. Verifies employee via photo ID or company representative.		
3. Obtains appropriate form(s): • Chain of custody		
4. Verbalizes urine collection steps per Department of Transportation (DOT) Standards: • Healthcare provider and patient wash hands; healthcare provider wears appropriate PPE. • Room is secured with no water available. • Healthcare worker opens collection kit in front of employee. • Employee obtains urine specimen in collection cup. • Healthcare worker checks temperature. • Healthcare worker splits urine specimen into the 2 specimen containers and places tamper strips over containers. • Healthcare worker dates tamper strips. • Employee initials tamper strips after they are placed on the containers. • Specimens are placed in bag. • All areas of chain of custody are filled out, including company name, employee's social security number, collection site, employee ID'd by…, phone and fax number, temperature, split specimen, employee (donor) name and signature, Healthcare worker (collector) name and signature and specimen released to… • Healthcare worker keeps "collector" copy of chain of custody form in the employee's chart. All other copies of chain of custody are placed in specimen bag and bag is sealed and sent to lab.		

MS—Medical-Surgical

5. Verbalizes blood collection steps per infection control practice guidelines: • Healthcare provider wears appropriate PPE. • Site should be prepped with nonalcohol/betadine solution. • Blood specimen will be labeled and sealed in front of employee with tamper label placed around the blood tube top with the label on the stopper and glass. • Specimen is taken to lab.		
6. Procedure and patient response documented in patient care record including: • Observed urine collection. • Preparation used for blood collection. • Specimen labeled and sealed in front of employee. • Chain of evidence.		

Self-assessment	Evaluation/ validation methods	Levels	Type of validation	Comments
❏ Experienced ❏ Need practice ❏ Never done ❏ Not applicable (based on scope of practice)	❏ Verbal ❏ Demonstration/ observation ❏ Practical exercise ❏ Interactive class	❏ Beginner ❏ Intermediate ❏ Expert	❏ Orientation ❏ Annual ❏ Other _____	

_____   _____
Employee signature   ***Observer signature***

Reference:
United States Department of Transportation. *Best practices for DOT random drug and alcohol testing.* Office of the Secretary and Office of Drug and Alcohol Policy and Compliance.

MS—Medical-Surgical

Name: _____ Date: _____

Skill: Flex Pen® Patient Self-Administration

Steps	Completed	Comments
1. Two nurses check order for insulin, type, device, dosage, frequency.		
2. Wash hands.		
3. Have patient/designee state prescribed dose.		
4. **Before every dose of NovoLog®, mix 70/30: roll the Flex Pen® up and down so that the glass ball moves back and forth from one end of the insulin reservoir to the other. Do this at least 10 times. Repeat till insulin appears uniformly white and cloudy.** <u>There must be at least 12 units in the NovoLog® 70/30 pen to ensure even mixing. If there is less than 12 units in the device, discard.</u>		
5. Remove cap and wipe with alcohol swab.		
6. Place a new NovoFine® needle on the FlexPen® for each injection.		
7. **With Each Dose**, turn the dose dial to 2 units. Holding the FlexPen® up. Depress the button to expel any air. Look for a drop of insulin. If no drop appears after 6 air shots, do not use and call pharmacy.		
8. Dial in the ordered dose. Dial can be turned either up or down in either direction. When dialing, be careful not to push button as insulin may be ejected. Do not dial in a dose greater than in vial.		

9. Observe patient/designee preparation and self-administration
   a. Clean off injection site with alcohol.
   b. Choose appropriate site, and gently insert the needle into the skin.
   c. Press the large injection button all the way in.
   d. With the button pushed in, keep needle in skin for at least 6 seconds to ensure full dose has been delivered.
   e. Remove from skin with button depressed.		

10. The patient disposes of the nonsafety needle to ensure nurse safety: No recapping, no breaking of needle. Disposal at point of use.		
11. Replace outer cap only on FlexPen®.		
12. Provide patient teaching, reinforcing prior patient teaching as necessary. a. Reinforce prior patient teaching as necessary.		
13. Remove FlexPen® from bedside and store in medication drawer. Prior to use, store FlexPen® in refrigerator. Once in use, FlexPen® can be kept un-refrigerated for the following days: Novolog® 70/30 14 days & Novolog® 28 days.		
14. When empty, discard. Always properly dispose of needles.		

Self-assessment	Evaluation/ validation methods	Levels	Type of validation	Comments
❏ Experienced ❏ Need practice ❏ Never done ❏ Not applicable (based on scope of practice)	❏ Verbal ❏ Demonstration/ observation ❏ Practical exercise ❏ Interactive class	❏ Beginner ❏ Intermediate ❏ Expert	❏ Orientation ❏ Annual ❏ Other _____	

_____   _____
Employee signature   ***Observer signature***

Reference:
Asakura, T., et al. 2006. Handling and safety of two insulin injection pens (FlexPen® and OptiClik®) in insulin-naïve type 2 diabetic patients. *Diabetes* 55 (Supp. 1): A457.

MS—Medical-Surgical

Name: _____ Date: _____

Skill: **Gemstar Pump**

Steps	Completed	Comments
I. Pump Set-Up:		
1. Inserts 2 AA batteries into bottom of pump.		
2. Attaches tubing to pump.		
3. Ensures tubing is primed and air free.		
4. Reviews order sheet.		
5. Turn pump on.		
II. Pump Programming:		
1. Stops and unlocks pump.		
2. Select delivery mode.		
3. Select unit of measure (mg/ml or ml).		
4. Enter concentration, if applicable.		
5. Enter continuous rate.		
6. Program a loading dose, Yes or No.		
7. Enter bolus dose.		
8. Enter bolus lockout.		
9. Enter # of boluses per hour.		
10. Program container size.		
11. Do program review.		
12. Restarts pump.		
III. Bag Changing:		
1. Stops and unlock pump.		
2. Attaches bag.		
3. Programs new container.		
4. Do program review.		
5. Restart pump.		
6. Documents bag change.		
IV. Documentation: **A. On Medication Administration Record/PRN Medication**		
1. **When medication is initiated** record:		
a. Time		
b. Ambulatory Pump		

MS—Medical-Surgical

c. Type of narcotic		
d. Pain score		
e. Initials of two nurses		
2. **At End of Each Shift** record:		
a. Time		
b. Actual pump volume reading		
c. Amount for shift		
d. Pain score		
e. Initials of RN		
3. **When Bag is completed** record:		
a. Time		
b. Actual pump volume reading		
c. Actual amount infused since shift change		
d. Pain score		
e. Initials of nurse RN (when new bag is added, one must be nurse, may be LPN) **NOTE:** If bag is changed during the shift, two entries are required on MAR **EXCEPTION:** Critical Care Units may record on the Critical Care Flowsheet the actual pump volume reading at the end of the shift or when a bag is completed.		
4. **When patient is transferred to another area** record:		
a. Time		
b. Actual pump volume reading		
c. Amount patient has received during the sending unit's shift.		
d. Pain score		
e. Initials of nurses – 2 nurses from sending unit one must be RN validate amount. Two nurses, one may be an LPN, in the receiving unit will validate this amount upon arrival by initials on MAR OR one nurse from the sending and one from the receiving unit validate amount.		

Evidence-Based Competency Management for the Medical-Surgical Unit, Second Edition

MS—Medical-Surgical

5. **When therapy is discontinued** record:		
a. Time		
b. Actual pump volume reading		
c. Amount patient receiving during shift		
d. Pain score		
e. Initials of nurse		
B. On Interdisciplinary Plan of Care		
1. Patient/Significant other education regarding sue of Gemstar Pump		
2. Patient/Significant other response to teaching		
C. On Ongoing Nursing Assessment		
1. Document pain goal		
2. Document type of narcotic and effectiveness using the Words, Intensity, Location & Duration.		
3. Assess and record sedation levels ordered with **initiation** of pain management therapy. **NOTE:** Critical Care units document pain score every four hours on Critical Care Flowsheet.		
D. Graphics Record		
1. Record respiratory rates as ordered with initiation of PCA or with dose change.		
2. Record respiratory rate every 4 hours as ordered during maintenance of PCA.		
E. On Parenteral Fluid Record		
1. Document according to IV administration procedure section 1 page 16.		

Self-assessment	Evaluation/ validation methods	Levels	Type of validation	Comments
❏ Experienced ❏ Need practice ❏ Never done ❏ Not applicable (based on scope of practice)	❏ Verbal ❏ Demonstration/ observation ❏ Practical exercise ❏ Interactive class	❏ Beginner ❏ Intermediate ❏ Expert	❏ Orientation ❏ Annual ❏ Other _____	

_____ _____
Employee signature *Observer signature*

Reference:
Fertig, B., Martin, D., and Simmons, D. 1995. Therapy for diabetes. *Diabetes in America*. 2nd ed. Bethesda, MD: National Institutes of Health. 519-540.

MS—Medical-Surgical

Name: _____ Date: _____

Skill: Homegoing Instructions

Steps	Completed	Comments
1. Explains to patient a copy of the homegoing instructions forms and gives a copy to the patient/significant other upon discharge.		
2. Completely fills out each section of the homegoing instruction form.		
3. Uses patient language.		
4. Prints instructions firmly and legibly.		
5. Does not use abbreviations.		
6. Fits medication times into the patient's schedule.		
Medications:		
7. Documents all homegoing medications including • Name/strength/dose • Times to take		
8. Discusses all new medications with patient.		
9. Gives medication information sheet for all new medications and initials documentation.		
Special instructions/purpose		
10. Documents any special instructions, precautions, suggestions, and food/drug interactions.		
Diet instructions		
11. Appropriate box is checked.		
Activity/special restrictions		
12. Checks appropriate box is checked. If restrictions apply, documents specific restrictions.		
Call your doctor if:		
13. Writes any information or concerns for which the patient should call his or her physician in this section.		
Additional instructions/educational materials provided		
14. Documents reference material that the patient is to use at home.		
15. Instructions are clear and concise.		

16. Marks appropriate advance directives box, indicating information was given or patient has advance directives.		
Follow-up care/community resource follow-up		
17. Documents time and place of appointment and with whom.		
18. Documents physician or clinic appointments as well as any other community resource follow-up.		
Patient signature		
19. Patient or significant other signs in appropriate area upon discharge. If significant other signing, notes his or her relationship to patient.		
Discharge information		
20. Documents date, time, and mode of discharge. Marks appropriate box to indicate to where the patient is discharged.		
Signature/initial section		
21. Enters full signature and writes corresponding initials on the appropriate line when patient education is given.		

Self-assessment	Evaluation/ validation methods	Levels	Type of validation	Comments
❏ Experienced ❏ Need practice ❏ Never done ❏ Not applicable (based on scope of practice)	❏ Verbal ❏ Demonstration/ observation ❏ Practical exercise ❏ Interactive class	❏ Beginner ❏ Intermediate ❏ Expert	❏ Orientation ❏ Annual ❏ Other _____	

_____   _____

Employee signature   *Observer signature*

Reference:
Duell, D., Martin, B., and Smith, S. 2008. *Clinical Nursing Skills: Basic to Advanced Skills*. 7th ed. Upper Saddle River, NJ: Pearson Education, Inc.

MS—Medical-Surgical

Name: _____ Date: _____

Skill: Hypodermoclysis

Steps	Completed	Comments
1. Identify patient, provide for privacy.		
2. Sanitize hands. Put on gloves.		
3. Prep site with alcohol. Sites acceptable: • Abdomen • Anterior or lateral thigh		
4. Carefully remove the Aqua=C needle set from the plastic tube. (The undersurface of the set [needle side] has an adhesive backing with no liner.)		
5. Remove end cap on the spike and insert it into the solution container.		
6. Connect the Aqua=C to the 82" (20 drop) IV set.		
7. Suspend the solution container and prime the drip chamber and the Aqua=C needle set, until you can see drops from both needles of the Aqua=C.		
8. Close the flow regulator and insert the Aqua=C into the patient at the chosen site. • Remove the needle guard from the needle. • Grasp the needle set by the edge of the strip and insert needle into prepared site straight down at a 90 angle. • Lay the flexible body-conforming base flat against the site.		
9. Apply the transparent dressing provided.		
10. Set the flow regulator to the desired flow rate.		
11. Check drip chamber/flow regulator as necessary.		
12. If fluid accumulation under the skin is observed, slow flow rate to allow for fluid dispersion.		
MAINTENANCE		
1. Rotate infusion sites with each liter of fluid or at the first sign of pain, redness, swelling or leakage at the site.		

2. Assess the infusion site at least once every four hours for redness, swelling and/or pain, leaking or dislodged needle. Change site as clinically indicated. Document observations on Nursing Progress Record.

3. Change site every liter of fluid.

4. Changes or distress notify the most physician/delegate.

REMOVAL OF AQUA=C

EQUIPMENT
   a. Nonsterile gloves
   b. 3"x3" gauze square
   c. Band-aid

PERFORMANCE PHASE

1. Check MD order.
2. Wash hands, put on gloves.
3. Stop the infusion when complete.
4. Remove the tape over the tubing loops and remove the dressing.
5. Remove the disk by pulling it straight out.
6. Apply pressure to the insertion site if fluid leakage is present.
7. Cleanse the area with N/S and cover the site with a small sterile dressing.
8. Dispose of all used equipment and supplies in an appropriate manner.

Self-assessment	Evaluation/ validation methods	Levels	Type of validation	Comments
❏ Experienced ❏ Need practice ❏ Never done ❏ Not applicable (based on scope of practice)	❏ Verbal ❏ Demonstration/ observation ❏ Practical exercise ❏ Interactive class	❏ Beginner ❏ Intermediate ❏ Expert	❏ Orientation ❏ Annual ❏ Other _____	

Employee signature   *Observer signature*

Reference:
Norfolk Medical Products, Inc. 2003. Aqua-C Hydration System Resource Guide. Skokie, IL: Norfolk Medical Products, Inc.

Sasson, M. and Shvartzman, P. 2001. Hypodermoclysis: An alternative infusion technique. *American Family Physician* 64(9): 1575-1578.

MS—Medical-Surgical

Name: _____   Date: _____

Skill: Infusion Intravenous Piggyback Antibiotics (IVPB)

Steps	Completed	Comments
1. Washes hands.		
2. Reviews physician's orders.		
3. Assembles equipment.		
• Mini bag antibiotics — checks patient's name against name on mini bag, expiration date, volume of rate.		
• Secondary IV tubing.		
• Alcohol swab.		
4. Explains procedure to patient.		
5. Attaches secondary IV tubing to mini bag:		
• Back flushing — if this is not first dose.		
• Holds secondary IVPB bag below level of primary IV bag and allows some of primary fluid to flow into line and "used" IVPB.		
• Clamps secondary line.		
• Removes old IVPB bag.		
• Attaches next IVPB to be infused.		
6. Hangs primary bag on hook lower than secondary bag.		
7. Opens secondary clamp and infuse IVPB.		
8. Program pump:		
• Secondary volume to be infused is to equal volume of IVPB.		
• Rate to be infused is rate to deliver IVPB antibiotics in time indicated on bag.		
9. Returns pump to primary rate to be infused when IVPB is complete.		
10. Documents IVPB antibiotic on MAR.		

MS—Medical-Surgical

Self-assessment	Evaluation/ validation methods	Levels	Type of validation	Comments
❏ Experienced ❏ Need practice ❏ Never done ❏ Not applicable (based on scope of practice)	❏ Verbal ❏ Demonstration/ observation ❏ Practical exercise ❏ Interactive class	❏ Beginner ❏ Intermediate ❏ Expert	❏ Orientation ❏ Annual ❏ Other _____	

_____   _____
Employee signature   *Observer signature*

Reference:
Weinstein, S. 2007. *Plumer's Principles and Practice of Intravenous Therapy*. 8th ed. Philadelphia, PA: Lippincott.

MS—Medical-Surgical

Name: _____ Date: _____

Skill: **Inline Tracheobronchial Suctioning**

Steps	Completed	Comments
1. Introduces self.		
2. Explains procedure.		
3. Ensures privacy.		
4. Washes hands.		
5. Positions patient in semi- or high-Fowler's position.		
6. Auscultates lung sounds.		
7. Preoxygenates patient.		
8. Turns inline suction regulator to open position.		
9. Advances inline catheter into tracheobronchial tree.		
10. Applies suction by compressing inline suction regulator with thumb and withdraws catheter, taking no more than 15 seconds.		
11. Monitors cardiac status.		
12. Clears suction catheter by instilling sterile NS into instillation port while applying continuous suction with thumb, compressing inline suction regular.		
13. Turns inline regulator to locked position.		
14. Postoxygenates patient.		
15. Repeats Steps 7, 8, 9, 10, 11, and 12 as necessary.		
16. Auscultates lung sounds.		
17. Washes hands.		
18. Documents procedure and sputum characteristics in nurse's notes.		
19. Routine NS irrigation is not recommended!		

Self-assessment	Evaluation/ validation methods	Levels	Type of validation	Comments
❏ Experienced ❏ Need practice ❏ Never done ❏ Not applicable (based on scope of practice)	❏ Verbal ❏ Demonstration/ observation ❏ Practical exercise ❏ Interactive class	❏ Beginner ❏ Intermediate ❏ Expert	❏ Orientation ❏ Annual ❏ Other _____	

_____   _____
Employee signature   *Observer signature*

Reference:
Carlson, K. and Weigand, D. 2005. *AACN Procedure Manual for Critical Care*. 5th ed. St. Louis, MO: Elsevier Saunders. 62-69.

MS—Medical-Surgical

Name: _____ Date: _____

Skill: Insertion of Dobbhoff Feeding Tube

Steps	Completed	Comments
1. Assembles equipment • Dobbhoff ® feeding tube with stylet • 60-cc luer tip syringe • Flashlight/pen light • Tape • Water soluble lubricant • Nonsterile gloves • Towel • Pulse oximeter • Tincture of benzoin of liquid adhesive • Permanent marking pen		
2. Explains procedure to patient.		
3. Positions patient in high-Fowler's position.		
4. Drapes patient and places pulse oximeter on patient.		
5. Washes hands and dons gloves.		
6. Checks feeding tube for flaws.		
7. Measures distance to insert gastric tube and marks tube with pen.		
8. Submerges tip of tube into water for five seconds to activate lubricant.		
9. For duodenal placement: places a 30° bend in tube and stylet approximately 6 cm from end of tube.		
10. Inserts feeding tube into nasopharynx and advances into oropharynx.		
11. Advances tube into esophagus, using sips of water if not contraindicated.		
12. Advances tube to premeasured mark.		
13. Confirms gastric placement of injecting 15 mL bursts of air while auscultating LUQ, epigastrium, RUQ, and RLQ.		
14. If duodenal placement is ordered, lowers HOB to <15° and places patient on R side • Advances tube additional 25 cm while injecting 5 mL bursts of air.		

15. Confirms duodenal placement by auscultation.		
16. Cleanses secretions and lubricant from external portion of feeding tube and patient's nose.		
17. Applies tincture of benzoin to 2–3 inches of external feeding tube and to top of the patient's nose.		
17. Applies tincture of benzoin to 2–3 inches of external feeding tube and to top of patient's nose.		
18. Tapes tube securely to nose/cheek with tape.		
19. Marks tube at exit from nares with permanent marking pen.		
20. Obtains appropriate x-ray.		
21. Pulls out stylet when radiographic confirmation is obtained.		
22. Documents procedure on appropriate forms.		

Self-assessment	Evaluation/ validation methods	Levels	Type of validation	Comments
❏ Experienced ❏ Need practice ❏ Never done ❏ Not applicable (based on scope of practice)	❏ Verbal ❏ Demonstration/ observation ❏ Practical exercise ❏ Interactive class	❏ Beginner ❏ Intermediate ❏ Expert	❏ Orientation ❏ Annual ❏ Other _____	

_____ _____
Employee signature   **Observer signature**

Reference:
Weinstein, S. 2007. *Plumer's Principles and Practice of Intravenous Therapy*. 8th ed. Philadelphia, PA: Lippincott.

MS—Medical-Surgical

Name: _____ Date: _____

Skill: Insulin Administration

Steps	Completed	Comments

1. Check preparation with another nurse.
  a. Physician's order sheets are reviewed from the current date back to the most recent written insulin order to ensure accuracy.
  b. Check the label to verify source, type, concentration, and expiration date of the insulin. **Note:** Pharmacy may be substituting brands of insulin.
  c. Verify dosage by drawing insulin(s) into syringe in the presence of a second nurse. For teaching purposes, after verification of dose and type of insulin, the nurse and patient may verify the filled syringe.
  d. Both nurses are to initial the Diabetes Flow Sheet in area provided. The RN can initial "per MD" if the physician is the second person checking the dose.		

2. Identify the patient by checking the following: a. Patient name and medical record number/birth date on identification band with patient name and medical record number on MAR.		

3. Identifies sites of injection. The preferred injection area is the abdominal region.
  a. To locate the abdominal sites, place two finger breadths away from the umbilicus, and begin injection rotation.
  b. All injections in the same anatomical area to be given at least 1 inch apart.
  c. If patient is on both **SQ insulin and SQ heparin**, the heparin is administered into the abdominal region. If necessary, insulin may be administered in another anatomical site (ex: thigh, upper arm, buttocks). Avoid ecchymotic areas.
  d. When rotating injection sites, (to areas other than the abdomen) use one area only, until it is used up.		

MS—Medical-Surgical

4. Give medication subcutaneously unless other wise indicated by the physician, and observe these guidelines:
   a. Perform hand hygiene and apply disposable gloves
   b. Clean skin with antiseptic
   c. Gently pinch or spread skin
   d. Insert needle into the skin at 90° angle
   e. Do not aspirate
   f. Do not massage
   g. Rotate injection sites in abdominal region.		

5. Disposes of sharps, remove gloves and perform hand hygiene.		
6. Documents on MAR and Diabetic Flow Sheet.		

Self-assessment	Evaluation/ validation methods	Levels	Type of validation	Comments
❏ Experienced ❏ Need practice ❏ Never done ❏ Not applicable (based on scope of practice)	❏ Verbal ❏ Demonstration/ observation ❏ Practical exercise ❏ Interactive class	❏ Beginner ❏ Intermediate ❏ Expert	❏ Orientation ❏ Annual ❏ Other _____	

_____   _____
Employee signature   *Observer signature*

Reference:
American Diabetes Association. 2003. Position statement on insulin administration. *Diabetes Care* 26(Supp. 1): 121.

Perry, A. and Potter, P. 2006. *Clinical Nursing Skills & Techniques.* 6th ed. St. Louis, MO: Mosby Elsevier.

Evidence-Based Competency Management for the Medical-Surgical Unit, Second Edition

MS—Medical-Surgical

Name: _____ Date: _____

Skill: **Insulin Administration Instruction**

Steps	Completed	Comments
1. Obtains equipment: getting started kit, practice bottle(s), of insulin(s), insulin guide(s), alcohol wipe, appropriate syringe size, bottle of sterile normal saline, syringe disposal guide, hypoglycemia handout, abdominal site rotation, glucose tablets. Instructs patient to wash hands. Explains how to read syringe and parts of syringe.		
2. Identifies and describes procedure for drawing up single or mixed insulin to patient via demonstration.		
3. Instructs patient to draw up at least two practice doses of insulin, using prescribed doses.		
4. Instructs patient on self-injecting technique into abdomen.		
5. Instructs patient on abdominal site rotation pattern, or other site as indicated.		
6. Instructs patient on proper disposal of needle and syringe.		
7. Instructs patient in symptoms, treatment, and prevention of hypoglycemia.		
8. Instructs patient in meal timing to correlate with insulin administration and to prevent hypoglycemia.		
9. Instructs patient in insulin source type, dose, and time of administration.		
10. Instructs patients in storage of insulin. (Store open vial of insulin at room temperature for 30 days, then discard. Refrigerate unopened vial of insulin according to manufacturer's directions.)		

11. Documents all steps of patient's performance R/T insulin administration.
    a. Inpatient forms.
    b. Makes referrals according to patient's needs.		

MS—Medical-Surgical

Self-assessment	Evaluation/ validation methods	Levels	Type of validation	Comments
❏ Experienced ❏ Need practice ❏ Never done ❏ Not applicable (based on scope of practice)	❏ Verbal ❏ Demonstration/ observation ❏ Practical exercise ❏ Interactive class	❏ Beginner ❏ Intermediate ❏ Expert	❏ Orientation ❏ Annual ❏ Other _____	

Employee signature

Observer signature

Reference:
American Diabetes Association. 2003. Position statement on insulin administration. *Diabetes Care* 26(Supp. 1): 121.

Perry, A. and Potter, P. 2006. *Clinical Nursing Skills & Techniques.* 6th ed. St. Louis, MO: Mosby Elsevier.

MS—Medical-Surgical

Name: _____ Date: _____

Skill: **Intramuscular Injections**

Steps	Completed	Comments
1. Identifies the three sites commonly used for IM medications.		
2. Verbalizes the five rights of medication administration.		
3. Demonstrates the skill in administering an IM medication.		
4. Explains the Z-track method of IM medication.		
5. Verbalizes the amount of medication that can be administered in an injection site.		
Pediatric:		
1. Identifies appropriate injection site for children under three years of age.		
2. Identifies appropriate injection site for children over three years of age.		
3. Verbalizes the amount of medication that can be administered in one injection site.		

Self-assessment	Evaluation/ validation methods	Levels	Type of validation	Comments
❏ Experienced ❏ Need practice ❏ Never done ❏ Not applicable (based on scope of practice)	❏ Verbal ❏ Demonstration/ observation ❏ Practical exercise ❏ Interactive class	❏ Beginner ❏ Intermediate ❏ Expert	❏ Orientation ❏ Annual ❏ Other _____	

_____   _____
Employee signature   *Observer signature*

Reference:
Duell, D., Martin, B., and Smith, S. 2008. *Clinical Nursing Skills: Basic to Advanced Skills.* 7th ed. Upper Saddle River, NJ: Pearson Education, Inc.

MS—Medical-Surgical

Name: _____ Date: _____

Skill: Intravenous Catheters—Declotting

Steps	Completed	Comments
1. Obtain appropriate equipment: 3 way stopcock, 10 cc syringe, 3 cc syringe and declotting agent.		
2. Explain procedure to patient.		
3. Position patient.		
4. Sanitize hands, using sterile technique apply stopcock directly to catheter with arrow pointed off toward catheter.		
5. Attach empty 10 cc syringe at 6:00 position.		
6. Attach 10 cc syringes with declotting agent at 3:00 position.		
7. Turn off key to 3:00 position and pull on the empty 10 cc syringe to create negative pressure.		
8. While maintaining negative pressure, turn off key toward 10 cc syringe. (This will pull required amount of declotting agent into catheter).		
9. Wait at least 15 minutes.		
10. Point turn off key to 3:00 and attempt to withdraw blood by pulling back on 10 cc syringe.		
11. If unsuccessful repeat steps 4 and 5.		
12. If a blood return is achieved withdraw 6 ml of blood.		
13. Flush with 20 ml of N/S followed by amount of heparin required for the line.		

Self-assessment	Evaluation/ validation methods	Levels	Type of validation	Comments
❏ Experienced ❏ Need practice ❏ Never done ❏ Not applicable (based on scope of practice)	❏ Verbal ❏ Demonstration/ observation ❏ Practical exercise ❏ Interactive class	❏ Beginner ❏ Intermediate ❏ Expert	❏ Orientation ❏ Annual ❏ Other _____	

_____   _____
Employee signature   **Observer signature**

Reference:
Weinstein, S. 2007. *Plumer's Principles and Practice of Intravenous Therapy*. 8th ed. Philadelphia, PA: Lippincott.

MS—Medical-Surgical

Name: _____ Date: _____

Skill: IV Dressing Changes

Steps	Completed	Comments
1. Evaluates need to change dressing.		
a. Time frame.		
b. Condition – Intactness – Dryness		
2. Assembles equipment.		
a. Sterile 2x2 or transparent dressing		
b. Prep swabs		
c. Gloves		
3. Explains procedure.		
4. Washes hands. Dons gloves.		
5. Removes tape, gauze/transparent dressing one layer at a time.		
6. Stabilizes catheter/needle with one hand, removing tape with other hand. (Does not lose contact with site.)		
7. Cleanses adhesive tape off site.		
8. Cleanses site with prep swabs.		
9. Replaces single strip of tape as appropriate to anchor catheter or tape over needle. Doesn't tape over insertion site.		
10. Places dressing over venipuncture site, tapes.		
11. Anchors tubing.		
12. Labels IV dressing.		
13. Records procedure and findings.		

Self-assessment	Evaluation/ validation methods	Levels	Type of validation	Comments
❏ Experienced ❏ Need practice ❏ Never done ❏ Not applicable (based on scope of practice)	❏ Verbal ❏ Demonstration/ observation ❏ Practical exercise ❏ Interactive class	❏ Beginner ❏ Intermediate ❏ Expert	❏ Orientation ❏ Annual ❏ Other _____	

_____   _____

Employee signature   *Observer signature*

Reference:
Weinstein, S. 2007. *Plumer's Principles and Practice of Intravenous Therapy*. 8th ed. Philadelphia, PA: Lippincott.

MS—Medical-Surgical

Name: _____ Date: _____

Skill: IV Site—Drawing Blood

Steps	Completed	Comments
1. Using personal protective equipment, inserts Insyte catheter in usual manner.		
2. Removes stylette (needle).		
3. Leaves tourniquet in place.		
4. Attaches "multiple sample" luer adapter to vacutainer.		
5. Inserts vacutainer into Insyte and changes blood tubes as needed for ordered blood specimens.		
6. Removes tourniquet.		
7. Removes vacutainer.		
8. Inserts IV tubing.		

Self-assessment	Evaluation/ validation methods	Levels	Type of validation	Comments
❏ Experienced ❏ Need practice ❏ Never done ❏ Not applicable (based on scope of practice)	❏ Verbal ❏ Demonstration/ observation ❏ Practical exercise ❏ Interactive class	❏ Beginner ❏ Intermediate ❏ Expert	❏ Orientation ❏ Annual ❏ Other _____	

_____   _____
Employee signature   *Observer signature*

Reference:
McCall, R. and Tankersley, C. 2007. *Phlebotomy Essentials*. 4th ed. Philadelphia, PA: Lippincott Williams & Wilkins.

MS—Medical-Surgical

Name: _____ Date: _____

Skill: IV Start—Hemodialysis Catheter

Steps	Completed	Comments
A. Obtains blood samples from IV catheter.		
1. Verbalizes policy for nonhemodialysis use of catheter. Must have Nephrologist order to access. Must be nephrology nurse.		
2. Gathers supplies: sterile gauze, gloves (sterile), mask, 10cc syringe, alcohol pad, primed IV tubing on pump.		
3. Determines priming volume of catheter port to be used for sampling.		
4. Identifies patient using two identifiers.		
5. Explains procedure to patient.		
6. Puts on gloves and mask.		
7. Removes tape if present from port to be used.		
8. Prepares a sterile gauze under catheter limb.		
9. With alcohol cleanse catheter blue venous port using friction.		
10. Confirms port clamp closed then removes and discards PRN adapter. Explains rationale for having catheter clamp closed when port opened and exposed to atmospheric air.		
11. Explains immediate nursing action in the event air is introduced into the catheter.		
12. Using 10cc syringe aspirates and discards heparin from open limb using 3 cc syringe. **Explain procedure if unable to obtain blood.		
13. Obtains blood samples – use second 10cc syringe.		
14. Flushes limb with 10 cc of N/S w/o preservative with new 10cc syringe. No IV – go to step 17.		
IV Start: 15. Connect IV solution and program pump, open clamp. • Start IV		

Evidence-Based Competency Management for the Medical-Surgical Unit, Second Edition

MS—Medical-Surgical

16. Stop infusion.		
17. Clamp limb and connect 10 cc syringe.		
18. Instills heparin 1:1000 to priming volume of limb (instills rapidly and clamps while syringe plunger still moving forward).		
19. Recaps limb using new sterile PRN adapter (primed as needed).		
20. Secures PRN adapter with tape.		
21. Wraps limbs with gauze.		

Self-assessment	Evaluation/ validation methods	Levels	Type of validation	Comments
❑ Experienced ❑ Need practice ❑ Never done ❑ Not applicable (based on scope of practice)	❑ Verbal ❑ Demonstration/ observation ❑ Practical exercise ❑ Interactive class	❑ Beginner ❑ Intermediate ❑ Expert	❑ Orientation ❑ Annual ❑ Other _____	

_____   _____
Employee signature   *Observer signature*

Reference:
National Kidney Foundation. *Clinical Practice Guidelines.* www.kidney.org/professionals/doqi/guidelines/doqiupvai.html#doqiupva3 (accessed January 2007).

MS—Medical-Surgical

Name: _____ Date: _____

Skill: IV Starts and PRN Adapter

Steps	Completed	Comments
IV starts		
1. Identifies IV orders for: • Solution • Amount • Medication • Rate of flow		
2. Assesses site.		
3. Prepares IV equipment.		
4. Uses BSI technique/protection.		
5. Cleanses site with alcohol.		
6. Inserts appropriate needle/catheter.		
7. Applies appropriate dressing.		
8. States what to document relating to IV starts.		
PRN adapter		
1. Primes PRN adapter.		
2. Attaches sterile primed PRN adapter to hub of catheter.		
3. Cleans latex port of PRN adapter and injects with 22 cc N/S.		
4. Verbalizes how to check patency and sequence for administering medications via PRN adapter.		

Self-assessment	Evaluation/validation methods	Levels	Type of validation	Comments
❏ Experienced ❏ Need practice ❏ Never done ❏ Not applicable (based on scope of practice)	❏ Verbal ❏ Demonstration/observation ❏ Practical exercise ❏ Interactive class	❏ Beginner ❏ Intermediate ❏ Expert	❏ Orientation ❏ Annual ❏ Other _____	

_____ _____
Employee signature   *Observer signature*

Reference:
Weinstein, S. 2007. *Plumer's Principles and Practice of Intravenous Therapy*. 8th ed. Philadelphia, PA: Lippincott.

MS—Medical-Surgical

Name: _____ Date: _____

Skill: IV Therapy Documentation

Steps	Completed	Comments
Initiation documentation		
1. Time of insertion.		
2. Type of solution/amount.		
3. Rate of infusion.		
4. Location of insertion site.		
5. Type, gauge of needle/catheter.		
6. Patient response.		
7. Condition site.		
Maintenance documentation		
1. Time.		
2. Location of site.		
3. Solution/rate.		
4. Solution change.		
5. Tubing change.		
6. Site care/dressing.		
7. Condition of site/skin.		
8. Patient response.		
9. Fluid balance.		
Conversion documentation		
1. Time.		
2. Location of insertion site.		
3. Type/gauge of needle/catheter.		
4. Type/amount of solution.		
5. Condition of site/skin.		
6. Site care/dressing.		
7. Amount/type of flush solution and effectiveness of flush.		
8. Patient response.		
9. Fluid balance.		
Discontinuation documentation		
1. Time.		
2. Type/gauge of needle/catheter.		

3. Condition of skin/site.		
4. Patient response.		
5. Fluid balance.		
6. Condition of needle/catheter.		

Self-assessment	Evaluation/ validation methods	Levels	Type of validation	Comments
❏ Experienced ❏ Need practice ❏ Never done ❏ Not applicable (based on scope of practice)	❏ Verbal ❏ Demonstration/ observation ❏ Practical exercise ❏ Interactive class	❏ Beginner ❏ Intermediate ❏ Expert	❏ Orientation ❏ Annual ❏ Other _____	

_____ _____
Employee signature   **Observer signature**

Reference:
Weinstein, S. 2007. *Plumer's Principles and Practice of Intravenous Therapy.* 8th ed. Philadelphia, PA: Lippincott.

MS—Medical-Surgical

Name: _____ Date: _____

Skill: **Lab Specimen Labeling Compliance**

Steps	Completed	Comments
1. Obtains appropriate equipment, labels, and requisitions.		
2. Identifies self and explains procedure and purpose.		
3. Assesses/selects appropriate venous site.		
4. Draws specimen according to BSI, policy, and procedure.		
5. Disposes of equipment according to BSI, P&P.		
6. Uses label specific for T&S/T&C.		
7. Labels blood specimen appropriately while viewing patient's identification band.		
8. Before leaving the bedside, two persons sign label and requisition to verify identity of patient and specimen.		

Self-assessment	Evaluation/ validation methods	Levels	Type of validation	Comments
❑ Experienced ❑ Need practice ❑ Never done ❑ Not applicable (based on scope of practice)	❑ Verbal ❑ Demonstration/ observation ❑ Practical exercise ❑ Interactive class	❑ Beginner ❑ Intermediate ❑ Expert	❑ Orientation ❑ Annual ❑ Other _____	

_____   _____
Employee signature   *Observer signature*

Reference:
Wiseman, J. 1998. *Standard Procedures for the Collection of Diagnostic Blood Specimens by Venipuncture.* 4th ed. Wayne, PA: National Committee for Clinical Laboratory Standards.

Name: _____ Date: _____

Skill: Lidocaine for Insertion of IV Catheters

Steps	Completed	Comments
1. Identify IV order.		

2. Assess patient for contraindications:
  a. "Caine" allergies
  b. Taking MAO inhibitors
  c. Liver failure		

3. Inform the patient of the use of a local anesthetic. The patient may refuse to have anesthetic used.		
4. Wash hands/wear gloves.		
5. Assess IV site.		
6. Prepare syringe with 0.1 ml of 1% Lidocaine.		
7. Prep the site with alcohol.		
8. Make a bleb contiguous with vein.		
9. Wait 25 seconds.		
10. Proceed with IV start as usual.		
11. Document use of Lidocaine and IV start.		

Self-assessment	Evaluation/ validation methods	Levels	Type of validation	Comments
❏ Experienced ❏ Need practice ❏ Never done ❏ Not applicable (based on scope of practice)	❏ Verbal ❏ Demonstration/ observation ❏ Practical exercise ❏ Interactive class	❏ Beginner ❏ Intermediate ❏ Expert	❏ Orientation ❏ Annual ❏ Other _____	

_____   _____
Employee signature   *Observer signature*

Reference:
Oncology Nursing Society (ONS). 2004. *Access device guidelines: recommendations for nursing practice and education.* 2nd ed. Pittsburgh, PA: Oncology Nursing Society.

MS—Medical-Surgical

Name: _____ Date: _____

Skill: **Maintenance of Hickman Catheter**

Steps	Completed	Comments
1. Gathers necessary equipment: • Clave adapter – 1 per lumen • Alcohol wipe — one per lumen • 10 cc syringe — two for each lumen • Heparinized saline (100 units/cc) prefilled syringe.		
2. Washes hands, wears sterile gloves.		
PRN adapter changes:		
3. Changes Clave adapter q week and prn.		
4. Clamps individual catheter pigtail with slide clamp.		
5. Cleanses hub connection with alcohol wipe & attaches new Clave adapter.		
Flushing:		
6. Flushes with 5 ml N/S using 10-cc syringe.		
7. Follows N/S flush with 2.5 cc heparinized saline (100 units/cc) using a 10-cc syringe.		
8. Withdraws syringe from Clave adapter while flushing the last 0.5 cc.		
9. Leaves catheter unclamped when not in use.		
10. Documents appropriately.		

Self-assessment	Evaluation/ validation methods	Levels	Type of validation	Comments
❑ Experienced ❑ Need practice ❑ Never done ❑ Not applicable (based on scope of practice)	❑ Verbal ❑ Demonstration/ observation ❑ Practical exercise ❑ Interactive class	❑ Beginner ❑ Intermediate ❑ Expert	❑ Orientation ❑ Annual ❑ Other _____	

_____   _____
Employee signature   *Observer signature*

Reference:
Batirel, H., Lacin, T., Yildizeli, F., and Yuksel, M. 2004. Complications and management of long-term central venous access catheters and ports. *Journal of Vascular Access* 5(4): 174-178.

MS—Medical-Surgical

Name: _____ Date: _____

Skill: **Metered Dose Inhaler (MDI)**

Steps	Completed	Comments
1. Identifies, explains to, and positions the patient for MDI administration.		

2. Gives complete and thorough instructions on how to use an MDI.
    a. Without a spacer
        1. Open mouth
        2. Close mouth
    b. With a spacer		

3. Assesses the patient before and after administration.
    a. Heart rate
    b. Respiratory
    c. Breath sounds
    d. Peak expiratory flows (if giving a bronchodilator)		

4. Administers the medication using an MDI
    a. Without a spacer
    b. With a spacer		

5. Encourages and assists the patient to cough/clear airway.		
6. Documents the procedure in the patient's chart (progress notes).		

Self-assessment	Evaluation/validation methods	Levels	Type of validation	Comments
❏ Experienced ❏ Need practice ❏ Never done ❏ Not applicable (based on scope of practice)	❏ Verbal ❏ Demonstration/observation ❏ Practical exercise ❏ Interactive class	❏ Beginner ❏ Intermediate ❏ Expert	❏ Orientation ❏ Annual ❏ Other _____	

_____ _____
Employee signature *Observer signature*

Reference:
Perry, A. and Potter, P. 2006. *Clinical Nursing Skills & Techniques.* 6th ed. St. Louis, MO: Mosby Elsevier.

Evidence-Based Competency Management for the Medical-Surgical Unit, Second Edition

MS—Medical-Surgical

Name: _____ Date: _____

Skill: Nasogastric Tube Maintenance

Steps	Completed	Comments
1. Verbalizes procedure for insertion of nasogastric tube (RN only).		
2. Disconnects tube from suction to assure suction is working.		
3. Identifies appropriate gomco suction settings. Salem sump: low continuous 30–40 mg/Hg.		
4. Verbalizes technique involved in checking for residual. Gentle aspirations with 60-cc syringe.		
5. Relates policies regarding irrigations of nasogastric tubes. (LPNs are not permitted to irrigate N/G tubes on patients with active GI bleed or postoperative gastric surgery patient. May irrigate nonoperative patients. Nongastric surgery patients after 24 hours.)		
6. Checks tape every shift to assure that it is clean, dry, and secure.		
7. Assesses bowel function regularly.		
8. Inspects drainage for color, consistency, and amount. Records I&O.		

Self-assessment	Evaluation/ validation methods	Levels	Type of validation	Comments
❑ Experienced ❑ Need practice ❑ Never done ❑ Not applicable (based on scope of practice)	❑ Verbal ❑ Demonstration/ observation ❑ Practical exercise ❑ Interactive class	❑ Beginner ❑ Intermediate ❑ Expert	❑ Orientation ❑ Annual ❑ Other _____	

_____   _____
Employee signature   *Observer signature*

Reference:
Perry, A. and Potter, P. 2006. *Clinical Nursing Skills & Techniques.* 6th ed. St. Louis, MO: Mosby Elsevier.

Name: _____ Date: _____

Skill: Nasopharyngeal Suctioning

Steps	Completed	Comments
1. Introduces self.		
2. Explains procedure.		
3. Ensures privacy.		
4. Washes hands.		
5. Assembles equipment.		
6. Positions patient in semi- or high-Fowler's position.		
7. Auscultates lung sounds.		
8. Turns on wall suction.		
9. Opens N/S.		
10. Opens suction catheter kit.		
11. Squeezes lubricant onto sterile field.		
12. Puts on sterile gloves.		
13. Pours N/S.		
14. Attaches catheter to suction tubing.		
15. Draw N/S through catheter.		
16. Lubricates catheter with nondominate hand.		
17. Directs catheter gently and without suction into nares until lit passes initial curve of resistance.		
18. With patient inhaling and without suction, continues to gently advance catheter.		
19. Occludes thumb air vent and withdraws the catheter in a rotating/twisting names.		
20. Does not remove catheter till suctioning series finished.		
21. Oxygenates patient between passes of catheter.		
22. Flushes catheter and tubing with N/S.		
23. Checks nares for bleeding.		
24. Suctions oral cavity.		
25. Flushes catheter and tubing.		
26. Wraps catheter in glove.		
27. Disposes in red bag trash.		

MS—Medical-Surgical

28. Turns off wall suction.		
29. Auscultates lung sounds.		
30. Disposes of supplies.		

Self-assessment	Evaluation/ validation methods	Levels	Type of validation	Comments
❏ Experienced ❏ Need practice ❏ Never done ❏ Not applicable (based on scope of practice)	❏ Verbal ❏ Demonstration/ observation ❏ Practical exercise ❏ Interactive class	❏ Beginner ❏ Intermediate ❏ Expert	❏ Orientation ❏ Annual ❏ Other _____	

_____   _____

Employee signature   *Observer signature*

Reference:
Perry, A. and Potter, P. 2006. *Clinical Nursing Skills & Techniques.* 6th ed. St. Louis, MO: Mosby Elsevier.

Name: _____ Date: _____

Skill: **Neurological Assessment and Documentation**

Steps	Completed	Comments
1. Uses the coagulation/neurovascular flow sheet to document neurological assessment.		
2. Records date and time of assessment in each column.		
3. Initials appropriate blocks.		
4. Correctly observes and records pupil reaction according to symbols (0 = absent, + = sluggish, ++ = reacts normally), along with appropriate number indicating size/shape of pupil.		
5. Correctly observes and records appropriate box(es) for orientation.		
6. Correctly observes and records responses for glasgow scale.		
Best verbal responses: **5** – If the patient is oriented to time, place, and person. **4** – If the patient is able to converse, although not oriented to time, place, and person (i.e., "Where am I?"). **3** – If the patient speaks only in words or phrases that make little or no sense. **2** – If the patient responds with incomprehensible sounds such as groans. **1** – If patient does not respond verbally at all.		
Eye-opening responses: **4** – If the patient opens his eyes spontaneously when the nurse approaches. **3** – If the patient opens his eyes in response to speech (spoken/shouted). **2** – If the patient opens his eyes only in response to painful stimuli (digital squeezing around nail-beds of fingers). **1** – If patient does not open his eyes in response to painful stimuli.		

Evidence-Based Competency Management for the Medical-Surgical Unit, Second Edition

Best motor responses: **6** – If the patient can obey a simple command such as "lift your left hand off the bed." **5** – If the patient moves a limb to locate the painful stimuli applied to the head or trunk and attempts to remove the source. **4** – If the patient attempts to withdraw form the source of pain. **3** – If the patient flexes only his arms at the elbows and wrist in response to painful stimuli to the nailbeds (decorticate rigidity). **2** – If the patient extends his arm (straightens elbows) in response to painful stimuli. **1** – If the patient has no motor response to pain on any limb.		
7. Checks hand grasp/pedal pushes bilaterally.		
8. Correctly records hand grasp/pedal pushes noting strong, weak, absent.		
9. Observes and records speech pattern by placing code in appropriate box (WNL–within normal limits, G–Garbled, S–Slurred, M–Moan, N–None).		
10. Observes and records sensation (WNL–If sensation is within normal limits, Other–If other than WNL or there is a change).		
11. Observes and records pulses. Note (L) left or (R) right plus the type of pulse being checked in the space provided.		
12. Writes N/A for information not applicable to patient.		
13. Documents any changes and description in the interdisciplinary progress notes.		

MS—Medical-Surgical

Self-assessment	Evaluation/validation methods	Levels	Type of validation	Comments
❏ Experienced ❏ Need practice ❏ Never done ❏ Not applicable (based on scope of practice)	❏ Verbal ❏ Demonstration/observation ❏ Practical exercise ❏ Interactive class	❏ Beginner ❏ Intermediate ❏ Expert	❏ Orientation ❏ Annual ❏ Other _____	

_____ _____
Employee signature   *Observer signature*

Reference:
Duell, D., Martin, B., and Smith, S. 2008. *Clinical Nursing Skills: Basic to Advanced Skills*. 7th ed. Upper Saddle River, NJ: Pearson Education, Inc.

MS—Medical-Surgical

Name: _____ Date: _____

Skill: Neurovascular Status of the Spinal Unit

Steps	Completed	Comments
1. Explains procedure to patient.		
2. Uses techniques correctly and in appropriate order.		
A. Assesses motor mobility of patients extremities: • Check ROM and muscle strength • Bilateral • From foot to hip		
B. Assesses circulatory status: • Checking pulses • Bilateral • Foot and leg pulses • Temperature — bilaterally • Color — bilaterally		
C. Assesses sensation: • Bilaterally • From toe to hip by touch		
3. Documents findings on neurovascular assessment form and nurse's notes		
4. Documents any changes in nurse's notes.		
5. Verbalizes abnormal changes to be reported to physician.		

Self-assessment	Evaluation/ validation methods	Levels	Type of validation	Comments

❏ Experienced
❏ Need practice
❏ Never done
❏ Not applicable
  (based on scope of
  practice)
	❏ Verbal
	❏ Demonstration/
	  observation
	❏ Practical exercise
	❏ Interactive class
		❏ Beginner
		❏ Intermediate
		❏ Expert
			❏ Orientation
			❏ Annual
			❏ Other _____	

_____   _____
Employee signature   *Observer signature*

Reference:
Perry, A. and Potter, P. 2006. *Clinical Nursing Skills & Techniques.* 6th ed. St. Louis, MO: Mosby Elsevier.

MS—Medical-Surgical

Name: _____ Date: _____

Skill: Neutropenic Precautions

Steps	Completed	Comments
1. Identifies patient with 1,000 absolute neutrophil count as candidates for neutropenic precaution.		
2. Posts appropriate signage on room door.		
3. Instructs patient/family of restrictions: • No fresh fruits, vegetables, or live plants. • No contact with persons who have a communicable disease. • All people in contact with patient wash hands.		
4. Encourages patient to practice good personal hygiene: • Wash hands after voiding and bowel movements. • Daily bathing. • Mouth care after meals and at H.S.		
5. Identifies need to prevent trauma to patient's skin or mucous membranes: • Avoids invasive procedures, per rectum meds. • Prevents constipation. • Promotes tissue integrity.		
6. Encourages patients to C & BD and ambulates if able.		
7. Documents neutropenic precautions maintained and patient/family education.		

Self-assessment	Evaluation/ validation methods	Levels	Type of validation	Comments
❏ Experienced ❏ Need practice ❏ Never done ❏ Not applicable (based on scope of practice)	❏ Verbal ❏ Demonstration/ observation ❏ Practical exercise ❏ Interactive class	❏ Beginner ❏ Intermediate ❏ Expert	❏ Orientation ❏ Annual ❏ Other _____	

_____ _____
Employee signature   *Observer signature*

Reference:
Oncology Nursing Society. 2005. *Chemotherapy and biotherapy guidelines and recommendations for practice*. 2nd ed. Pittsburgh, PA: Oncology Nursing Society.

MS—Medical-Surgical

Name: _____ Date: _____

Skill: NIH Stroke Scale, Completing the National Institutes of Health

Steps	Completed	Comments
1. Explains procedure to patient.		
2. Records performance in each category after each subscale exam.		

a. Level of consciousness
      • LOC questions
      • LOC commands.		

b. Best gaze.		
c. Visual.		
d. Facial palsy.		
e. Motor arm & leg.		
f. Limb ataxia.		
g. Sensory.		
h. Best language.		
i. Dysarthria.		
j. Extinction and inattention.		
3. Records answers while administering exam.		
4. Scores patient's first attempt.		
5. Enters total NIH stroke.		
6. Initials appropriate column and enters signature in block provided.		

Self-assessment	Evaluation/ validation methods	Levels	Type of validation	Comments
❏ Experienced ❏ Need practice ❏ Never done ❏ Not applicable (based on scope of practice)	❏ Verbal ❏ Demonstration/ observation ❏ Practical exercise ❏ Interactive class	❏ Beginner ❏ Intermediate ❏ Expert	❏ Orientation ❏ Annual ❏ Other _____	

_____ _____
Employee signature *Observer signature*

Reference:
National Institute of Health. National Institute of Neurological Disorders and Stroke. *http://www.ninds.nih.gov/index.htm* (accessed February 12, 2008).

Name: _____ Date: _____

Skill: **Normal Saline Wet to Dry Dressing**

Steps	Completed	Comments
1. Identifies order for wet-to-dry dressing change, noting site and frequency.		
2. Gathers supplies: clean gloves, sterile gloves, roller gauze (or wet to dry tin with roller gauze and 4x4s), 4x4s; noncotton, normal saline, sterile scissors, tape (or kerlix, or spandage). If packing deep/large wound, verifies with doctor the need for roller gauze; may choose to use kerlix or hand/burn gauze in place of 4x4s.		
3. Explains procedure to patient, offers pain med predressing change.		
4. Removes old dressing with clean gloves, removes slowly (reason for w-to-d is for debridement), if deep wound, removing too fast may cause more bleeding. (Removes all of old dressing, including string fragments of old gauze.)		
5. With sterile gloves on, cuts roller gauze to size of wound and places over open wound.		
6. Wets 4x4s with sterile normal saline, rings out to moderate dampness, and fluffs gauze piece to shape over roller gauze covering complete wound. Avoids placing damp gauze outside of wound (over good skin), thereby avoiding additional breakdown.		
7. Covers wet 4x4s with dry 4x4s		
8. Tapes into place or use kerlix or spandage PRN to prevent dressing from being displaced.		
9. Disposes of old dressing in red trash container.		
10. If set up sterile field to use again for frequent dressing changes, may use same field if kept covered and sterile for eight hours then discard.		

MS—Medical-Surgical

Self-assessment	Evaluation/ validation methods	Levels	Type of validation	Comments
❏ Experienced ❏ Need practice ❏ Never done ❏ Not applicable (based on scope of practice)	❏ Verbal ❏ Demonstration/ observation ❏ Practical exercise ❏ Interactive class	❏ Beginner ❏ Intermediate ❏ Expert	❏ Orientation ❏ Annual ❏ Other _____	

_____   _____
Employee signature   *Observer signature*

Reference:
Perry, A. and Potter, P. 2006. *Clinical Nursing Skills & Techniques.* 6th ed. St. Louis, MO: Mosby Elsevier.

MS—Medical-Surgical

Name: _____ Date: _____

Skill: **Ocular Medication Administration**

Steps	Completed	Comments
1. Identifies medication order: • Retina clinic, standing order • Review previous progress note upon assessment for "dilate on arrival" order • Dilating stamp • Locate physician order on medical record		
2. Demonstrates knowledge of asepsis: • Hand washing • Protection of sterility of eye dropper (medication bottle)		
3. Demonstrates appropriate steps of medication administration: • Identifies/verifies correct medication • Identifies patient • Identifies correct eye • Instills eye medication to inside of lower lid		
4. Demonstrates appropriate documentation per policy/procedure: • Documents time and initial/signature, as appropriate		
5. Demonstrates appropriate patient instruction regarding side effects of drops • Blurred near visual acuity for four to six hours • Photophobia • Offers sunglasses, as appropriate		
6. Demonstrates preservation of patient's privacy: • Protects medical record from viewing		

Self-assessment	Evaluation/validation methods	Levels	Type of validation	Comments
❏ Experienced ❏ Need practice ❏ Never done ❏ Not applicable (based on scope of practice)	❏ Verbal ❏ Demonstration/observation ❏ Practical exercise ❏ Interactive class	❏ Beginner ❏ Intermediate ❏ Expert	❏ Orientation ❏ Annual ❏ Other _____	

_____   _____
Employee signature   *Observer signature*

Reference:
Castaldi, P. 2005. *Clinical nursing skills and techniques.* 6th ed. St. Louis, MO: Elsevier Mosby.

Evidence-Based Competency Management for the Medical-Surgical Unit, Second Edition

MS—Medical-Surgical

Name: _____ Date: _____

Skill: **Ophthalmic Medication Administration**

Steps	Completed	Comments
General principles:		
1. Places date, time, and initials on multidose products when opening.		
2. Discards any products suspected of contamination.		
3. Discards ophthalmic preparations (drops, ointments, and solutions) according to expiration date.		
Medication administration:		
1. Reviews physician's medication order including drug name, concentration, number of drops (if a liquid), time, and eye (right or left) to receive medication.		
2. Checks client's identification by looking at identification bracelet and asking client's name.		
3. Washes hands.		
4. Explains procedure to client.		
5. Asks client to lie supine or sit back in chair with head slightly hyperextended.		
6. If crusts or drainage are present along eyelid margins or inner canthus, gently washes away. Soaks any crusts that are dried and difficult to remove by applying damp washcloth or cotton ball over eye for few minutes. Always wipes clean from inner to outer canthus.		
7. Holds cotton ball or clean tissue in nondominant hand just below lower eyelid.		
8. With tissue or cotton resting below lower lid, gently presses downward with thumb or forefinger against bony orbit.		
9. Asks client to look up toward ceiling.		

MS—Medical-Surgical

10. Instills eyedrops: 　A. Drops prescribed number of medication drops into conjunctival sac **(not onto cornea)**. 　B. If client blinks or closes eye, or if drops land on outer lid margins, repeats procedure. 　C. When administering drugs that cause systemic effects, protects finger with clean tissue and applies gentle pressure to clients nasolacrimal duct for 30–60 sec. 　D. After instilling drops, asks client to close eye gently.		
11. Instills eye ointment: 　A. Holding ointment applicator above lid margin, applies thin stream of ointment evenly along inside edge of lower eyelid on conjunctiva. 　B. Asks client to look down. 　C. Applies thin stream of ointment along upper lid margin on inner conjunctiva. 　D. Has client close eye and rub lid lightly in circular motion with cotton ball.		
12. If there is excess medication on eyelid, gently wipes it from inner to outer canthus.		
13. If client had eye patch, replaces it. Tapes securely without applying pressure to eye.		
14. Records received medication in medication administration record.		

Self-assessment	Evaluation/ validation methods	Levels	Type of validation	Comments
❏ Experienced ❏ Need practice ❏ Never done ❏ Not applicable (based on scope of practice)	❏ Verbal ❏ Demonstration/ observation ❏ Practical exercise ❏ Interactive class	❏ Beginner ❏ Intermediate ❏ Expert	❏ Orientation ❏ Annual ❏ Other _____	

_____   _____
Employee signature   *Observer signature*

Reference:
Duell, D., Martin, B., and Smith, S. 2008. *Clinical Nursing Skills: Basic to Advanced Skills.* 7th ed. Upper Saddle River, NJ: Pearson Education, Inc.

MS—Medical-Surgical

Name: _____ Date: _____

Skill: **Oral Care of the Cancer Patient**

Steps	Completed	Comments
1. Assembles equipment.		
2. Explains procedure to patient.		
3. Assesses oral cavity daily.		
4. Encourages use of routine oral hygiene regimen pc.		
• Uses soft sponge for mouth care as indicated.		
In patients with potential for stomatitis: • Rinses mouth 4x/day with 1 tsp. baking soda and 8 oz. water.		
• Uses soft foam toothbrush for tooth brushing.		
5. Applies topical anesthetics to mouth ac and prn as ordered.		
6. Documents procedure.		

Self-assessment	Evaluation/ validation methods	Levels	Type of validation	Comments
❏ Experienced ❏ Need practice ❏ Never done ❏ Not applicable (based on scope of practice)	❏ Verbal ❏ Demonstration/ observation ❏ Practical exercise ❏ Interactive class	❏ Beginner ❏ Intermediate ❏ Expert	❏ Orientation ❏ Annual ❏ Other _____	

_____   _____
Employee signature   *Observer signature*

Reference:
Perry, A. and Potter, P. 2006. *Clinical Nursing Skills & Techniques.* 6th ed. St. Louis, MO: Mosby Elsevier.

MS—Medical-Surgical

Name: _____ Date: _____

Skill: Patient-Controlled Analgesia (PCA) Infuser

Steps	Completed	Comments
1. Assembles PCA vial and injector.		
2. Connects vial to tubing and clears tubing.		
3. Prepares PCA infuser for insertion of vial.		
a. Turns on PCA pump		
b. Raises PCA drive assembly.		
4. Inserts vial.		
a. Checks for cracks		
5. Engages vial.		
a. Checks for proper placement		
6. Sets controls.		
a. Dose volume		
b. Lockout interval		
c. Loading dose		
7. Completes documentation.		

Self-assessment	Evaluation/ validation methods	Levels	Type of validation	Comments
❏ Experienced ❏ Need practice ❏ Never done ❏ Not applicable (based on scope of practice)	❏ Verbal ❏ Demonstration/ observation ❏ Practical exercise ❏ Interactive class	❏ Beginner ❏ Intermediate ❏ Expert	❏ Orientation ❏ Annual ❏ Other _____	

_____   _____

Employee signature   *Observer signature*

Reference:
Perry, A. and Potter, P. 2006. *Clinical Nursing Skills & Techniques.* 6th ed. St. Louis, MO: Mosby Elsevier.

MS—Medical-Surgical

Name: _____ Date: _____

Skill: Peripheral Blood Draw

Steps	Completed	Comments
1. Obtains appropriate equipment: requisition, vacutainer holder, blood tube(s), blood collection set, tourniquet, cotton balls, Band-Aid, gloves/personal protective equipment.		
2. Assesses/selects appropriate vein site (antecubital, forearm, or hand).		
3. Applies tourniquet 3–4 inches above the vein site with enough pressure to impede venous flow but not arterial flow.		
4. Instructs patient to open and close hand several times (distending veins).		
5. Prepares area with alcohol swab or providone-iodine swab. Allows to dry.		
6. Assembles vacutainer holder, blood collection set and tube(s).		
7. With bevel side up, introduces the butterfly needle into vein.		
8. Engages vacutainer tube by placing two fingers on the flange of the holder and gently pushing tube onto needle with thumb.		
9. Releases tourniquet as the last tube is filling (with multiple samples).		
10. When vacuum is exhausted and blood no longer flows, places a dry cotton ball over insertion site, withdraws needle from vein, and engages the safety shield.		
11. Applies pressure and Band-Aid to site.		
12. Disposes of equipment according to body substance isolation (BSI) requirements.		
13. Labels specimens at the bedside.		
14. Sends specimen(s) to appropriate lab.		
15. Documents procedure.		

Self-assessment	Evaluation/ validation methods	Levels	Type of validation	Comments
❑ Experienced ❑ Need practice ❑ Never done ❑ Not applicable (based on scope of practice)	❑ Verbal ❑ Demonstration/ observation ❑ Practical exercise ❑ Interactive class	❑ Beginner ❑ Intermediate ❑ Expert	❑ Orientation ❑ Annual ❑ Other _____	

_____ _____

Employee signature *Observer signature*

Reference:
Duell, D., Martin, B., and Smith, S. 2008. *Clinical Nursing Skills: Basic to Advanced Skills.* 7th ed. Upper Saddle River, NJ: Pearson Education, Inc.

Perry, A. and Potter, P. 2006. *Clinical Nursing Skills & Techniques.* 6th ed. St. Louis, MO: Mosby Elsevier.

MS—Medical-Surgical

Name: _____ Date: _____

Skill: PICC Line (Applying a PRN Adapter)

Steps	Completed	Comments
Registered nurse only Aseptic technique must be used during insertion, dressing changes, and any manipulation of the PICC.		
1. Applies a new CLC 2000 after initial insertion and then every week.		
2. Primes new CLC 2000 with normal saline.		
3. Vigorously cleans current connection of hub and CLC 2000 (if applicable).		
4. Removes used CLC 2000 and secures new one.		
5. Flushes with 5 mL of normal saline in a 10-cc syringe. When flushing, uses a pulsatile flush: quickly stop-start-stop-start while pushing on the plunger of the syringe.		
6. Flushes with 2.5 mL of heparin 1:100 units/mL if appropriate. When flushing, continues to inject the last 1/2 mL while at the same time withdrawing the syringe.		

Self-assessment	Evaluation/ validation methods	Levels	Type of validation	Comments
❏ Experienced ❏ Need practice ❏ Never done ❏ Not applicable (based on scope of practice)	❏ Verbal ❏ Demonstration/ observation ❏ Practical exercise ❏ Interactive class	❏ Beginner ❏ Intermediate ❏ Expert	❏ Orientation ❏ Annual ❏ Other _____	

_____ _____

Employee signature *Observer signature*

Reference:
Infusion Nurses Society. 2006. *Infusion Nursing Standards of Practice.* Norwood, MA: Infusion Nurses Society.

MS—Medical-Surgical

Name: _____ Date: _____

Skill: PICC Line (Obtaining Blood Samples)

Steps	Completed	Comments
Registered nurse only Aseptic technique must be used during insertion, dressing changes, and any manipulation of the PICC.		
1. Turns off IV 30 seconds prior to and while drawing blood.		
2. Clamps IV tubing and disconnects from PICC line. Does not permit air to enter line. Maintains sterility of disconnected IV line.		
3. Using 10-cc syringes:		
a. Flushes with 5 mL N/S.		
b. Withdraws 5 mL of blood for discard.		
c. Withdraws amount necessary for specimens.		
d. Flushes with 10 mL N/S. When flushing, uses a pulsatile flush quickly stop-start-stop-start while pushing on the plunger of the syringe.		
4. Reconnects the IV tubing, unclamps, and restarts infusion, or flushes with 2.5 mL heparin (100 u/mL). When flushing, continues to inject the last 1/2 mL while at the same time withdrawing the syringe.		
5. Sends specimen to lab and documents correctly.		

Self-assessment	Evaluation/validation methods	Levels	Type of validation	Comments
❏ Experienced ❏ Need practice ❏ Never done ❏ Not applicable (based on scope of practice)	❏ Verbal ❏ Demonstration/observation ❏ Practical exercise ❏ Interactive class	❏ Beginner ❏ Intermediate ❏ Expert	❏ Orientation ❏ Annual ❏ Other _____	

_____ _____
Employee signature *Observer signature*

Reference:
Infusion Nurses Society. 2006. *Infusion Nursing Standards of Practice.* Norwood, MA: Infusion Nurses Society.

MS—Medical-Surgical

Name: _____ Date: _____

Skill: PICC Line (Removing the PICC)

Steps	Completed	Comments
Registered nurse only Aseptic technique must be used during insertion, dressing changes, and any manipulation of the PICC.		
1. Requires aseptic technique, wears sterile gloves and mask.		
2. Carefully removes dressing.		
3. Removes sutures or steristrips.		
4. Places a folded 4x4 sponge over the insertion site but does not apply pressure.		
5. Slowly withdraws the PICC. Stops if any resistance is met. Waits a few minutes and attempts withdrawal again. If resistance continues, covers the site with a sterile dressing and notifies the physician or Nutrition Support Nurse.		
6. Applies betadine ointment and a 2x2 gauze dressing to site.		
7. Assesses condition and records length of PICC.		
8. Notifies physician of any noted abnormalities.		
9. Documents removal in interdisciplinary progress note: a. Date and time b. Condition of catheter and insertion site c. Culture, if ordered d. Patient tolerance e. Dressing application f. Instructions given to patient		

Self-assessment	Evaluation/ validation methods	Levels	Type of validation	Comments
❏ Experienced ❏ Need practice ❏ Never done ❏ Not applicable (based on scope of practice)	❏ Verbal ❏ Demonstration/ observation ❏ Practical exercise ❏ Interactive class	❏ Beginner ❏ Intermediate ❏ Expert	❏ Orientation ❏ Annual ❏ Other _____	

_____   _____
Employee signature   *Observer signature*

Reference:
Infusion Nurses Society. 2006. *Infusion Nursing Standards of Practice*. Norwood, MA: Infusion Nurses Society.

Name: _____ Date: _____

Skill: PICC Line (Starting and Discontinuing an Infusion)

Steps	Completed	Comments
Registered nurse only Aseptic technique must be used during insertion, dressing changes, and any manipulation of the PICC.		
A. Starting		
1. Prepares IV tubing with secure connection.		
2. Vigorously wipes PICC PRN adapter with an alcohol wipe.		
3. Using a 10-cc syringe, gently flushes the PICC with 5 mL of normal saline.		
4. If resistance is felt, checks PICC system for a closed clamp; if resistance persists, notify physician or nutrition support nurse.		
5. Cleans PRN adapter again with an alcohol wipe.		
6. Begins infusion. Secures IV tubing to PRN adapter, unclamps.		
7. If continuous infusion, connects hub to hub. Does not use PRN adapter.		
B. Discontinuing		
1. Clamps IV tubing and disconnects if from PRN adapter on PICC extension tubing.		
2. If discontinuing a continuous infusion, applies sterile PRN adapter to PICC or extension tubing on PICC.		
3. Cleans the PRN adapter vigorously with an alcohol wipe.		
4. Using 10-cc syringes:		
a. Flushes with 5 mL of normal saline. When flushing, uses a pulsatile flush: quickly stop-start-stop-start while pushing on the plunger of the syringe.		
b. Flushes with 2.5 mL of heparin 1:100 units/mL, withdrawing the needle while injecting the last 0.5 mL of heparin.		
C. Documentation		
1. Documents appropriately.		

MS—Medical-Surgical

Self-assessment	Evaluation/ validation methods	Levels	Type of validation	Comments
❏ Experienced ❏ Need practice ❏ Never done ❏ Not applicable (based on scope of practice)	❏ Verbal ❏ Demonstration/ observation ❏ Practical exercise ❏ Interactive class	❏ Beginner ❏ Intermediate ❏ Expert	❏ Orientation ❏ Annual ❏ Other _____	

_____
Employee signature

_____
Observer signature

Reference:
Infusion Nurses Society. 2006. *Infusion Nursing Standards of Practice.* Norwood, MA: Infusion Nurses Society.

MS—Medical-Surgical

Name: _____ Date: _____

Skill: **PICCS, Midlines and Central Lines—Suturing**

Steps	Completed	Comments
1. Utilize sterile technique.		
2. Visualizes proper positioning of PICC line tip.		
3. Numbs area to be sutured.		
4. Places suture in correct position in suture holder or penetration of skin.		
5. Penetrates skin superficially with suture and threads suture to exit skin in approximately one centimeter width.		
6. Ties triple knot so that the suture is loose from the skin.		
7. Wrap suture through wings of PICC line or through 2-3 times and tie a triple knot.		
8. Utilizes suture safety – not grabbing end of suture needle with fingers.		
9. Apply occlusive dressing.		

Self-assessment	Evaluation/ validation methods	Levels	Type of validation	Comments
❏ Experienced ❏ Need practice ❏ Never done ❏ Not applicable (based on scope of practice)	❏ Verbal ❏ Demonstration/ observation ❏ Practical exercise ❏ Interactive class	❏ Beginner ❏ Intermediate ❏ Expert	❏ Orientation ❏ Annual ❏ Other _____	

_____   _____
Employee signature   *Observer signature*

Reference:
Colyar, M. and Ehrhardt, C. 2001. *Ambulatory Care Procedures for the Nurse Practitioner*. Philadelphia, PA: F. A. Davis Company. 94-104.

Evidence-Based Competency Management for the Medical-Surgical Unit, Second Edition

MS—Medical-Surgical

Name: _____ Date: _____

Skill: Pin Care

Steps	Completed	Comments
1. Verifies physician order for pin care.		
2. Identifies patient and explains procedure.		
3. Identifies solutions and amount used.		
4. Pours equal amounts of 3 % H2O2 and normal saline in small sterile basin unless physician has ordered another solution.		
5. Places sterile applicators in basin.		
6. With a single applicator, cleanses area in a circular motion, starts at pin, and includes surrounding skin area. Pushes skin down to avoid skin growth around the pin.		
7. Repeats until all exudate is removed.		
8. Checks for loose pins. If found, report to physician.		
9. Inspects for signs of infection.		
10. Checks screws on pin. These must be tight.		
11. Leaves open to air unless otherwise ordered.		
12. Documents skin/pin site and patient education on chart.		
13. Marks appropriate billing sheet charge (ambulatory only).		

Self-assessment	Evaluation/ validation methods	Levels	Type of validation	Comments
❏ Experienced ❏ Need practice ❏ Never done ❏ Not applicable (based on scope of practice)	❏ Verbal ❏ Demonstration/ observation ❏ Practical exercise ❏ Interactive class	❏ Beginner ❏ Intermediate ❏ Expert	❏ Orientation ❏ Annual ❏ Other _____	

_____   _____
Employee signature   *Observer signature*

Reference:
National Association of Orthopaedic Nurses. *Guidelines for Orthopaedic Nursing.* www.orthonurse.org (accessed January 28, 2008).

MS—Medical-Surgical

Name: _____ Date: _____

Skill: **Postoperative Assessment**

Steps	Completed	Comments
Nursing care		
1. Assists in transfer of patient from PACU bed to own bed; makes comfortable, warm, and dry; raises side rails, bed to low position.		
2. Notes level of consciousness, skin condition, and color.		
3. Checks dressings and notes type and amount of drainage evident.		
4. Connects any drainage tubes to ordered devices.		
5. Records blood pressure, pulse, and respirations upon arrival to the unit; then every four hours x 48 hours; then every shift. Note: The physician or nurse may increase the frequency of vital signs based on assessment/reassessment data.		
6. Places call button within easy reach.		
7. Checks IV solution and prescribed flow rate.		
8. Notes appearance of IV site.		
9. Follows doctor's orders and performs postoperative routine nursing care.		
a. Intake: output for 24 hours or until all tubes removed.		
b. Administers pain medication as indicated. Checks anesthesia and PACU record for time, dose, and route of previously administered pain medication.		
c. Cough, deep breathe, and turn frequently unless contraindicated.		
d. Patients must be assisted by nursing personnel the first time out of bed.		
e. Any postoperative teaching specific to patient.		
Documentation		
A. Interdisciplinary plan of care/pathway		
1. Documents patient and significant other education and response to that education.		

Evidence-Based Competency Management for the Medical-Surgical Unit, Second Edition

MS—Medical-Surgical

a. Coughing and deep breathing exercises.		
b. Guarding incision.		
c. Pain control.		
B. Parenteral fluid record		
1. Documents according to IV administration procedure.		
C. Graphics/intake and output sheet		
1. Vital signs.		
2. Estimated blood loss.		
3. Intake and output (including bowel movement).		
4. SpO_2/FiO_2 if ordered.		
D. Interdisciplinary progress note		
1. Condition of patient on arrival to floor.		
2. Lack of progress toward goals.		
E. Ongoing nurse assessment		
1. Head-to-toe assessment.		

Self-assessment	Evaluation/ validation methods	Levels	Type of validation	Comments
❑ Experienced ❑ Need practice ❑ Never done ❑ Not applicable (based on scope of practice)	❑ Verbal ❑ Demonstration/ observation ❑ Practical exercise ❑ Interactive class	❑ Beginner ❑ Intermediate ❑ Expert	❑ Orientation ❑ Annual ❑ Other _____	

_____   _____
Employee signature   *Observer signature*

Reference:
Perry, A. and Potter, P. 2006. *Clinical Nursing Skills & Techniques.* 6th ed. St. Louis, MO: Mosby Elsevier.

MS—Medical-Surgical

Name: _____   Date: _____

Skill: Presenting a Patient at Team Rounds

Steps	Completed	Comments
New patient		
1. Reports or discusses each of the following		
a. Patient name		
b. Room number		
c. Physician		
d. Patients age		
e. Patients race		
f. Patients gender		
g. Admitting diagnosis		
h. Past medical history		
i. Medications prior to admission		
j. Nutritional status		
k. Hearing/sleep/vision		
l. Elimination		
m. Skin		
n. Memory		
o. Anxiety		
p. Depression		
q. Advanced directives		
r. DNR status		
s. Living arrangements		
t. Supports		
u. Current ADL		
v. Baseline ADL and IADL		
w. Treatment Plan		
x. ACE care plans (5 north only)		
y. Projected LOS		
z. Discharge plan		
Follow-up patient		
2. Reports or discusses each of the following		
a. Patient name		

Evidence-Based Competency Management for the Medical-Surgical Unit, Second Edition

MS—Medical-Surgical

b. Room number		
c. Physician		
d. Diagnosis		
e. New problems		
f. Current ADL's		
g. ACE care plans		
h. Projected LOS		
i. Discharge Plan		
j. Team suggestions		

Self-assessment	Evaluation/ validation methods	Levels	Type of validation	Comments
❏ Experienced ❏ Need practice ❏ Never done ❏ Not applicable (based on scope of practice)	❏ Verbal ❏ Demonstration/ observation ❏ Practical exercise ❏ Interactive class	❏ Beginner ❏ Intermediate ❏ Expert	❏ Orientation ❏ Annual ❏ Other _____	

_____   _____
Employee signature   *Observer signature*

Reference:
Perry, A. and Potter, P. 2006. *Clinical Nursing Skills & Techniques*. 6th ed. St. Louis, MO: Mosby Elsevier.

MS—Medical-Surgical

Name: _____ Date: _____

Skill: Pulse Oximeter Monitor

Steps	Completed	Comments
1. Verifies the physician's order for monitor.		
2. Washes hands.		
3. Obtains the appropriate equipment as required: a. Pulse oximeter b. Probe(s) c. Alcohol prep pads		
4. Identifies the patient and explains the procedure.		
5. Connects the power cord to 110v 60 Hz electrical outlet.		
6. Connects the oximeter probe to the monitor: a. Finger probe b. Ear probe c. Pediatric probe		
7. Turns on the power switch.		
8. Wipes the probe clean using an alcohol prep pad prior to applying it to the patient.		
9. Applies the probe to the patient's a. Finger b. Toe c. Ear d. Foot (infant)		
10. Observes for adequate wave form or pulse signal and reading.		
11. Sets alarm limits as required.		
12. Documents the procedure and initial reading in the patient's chart.		

Self-assessment	Evaluation/ validation methods	Levels	Type of validation	Comments
❏ Experienced ❏ Need practice ❏ Never done ❏ Not applicable (based on scope of practice)	❏ Verbal ❏ Demonstration/ observation ❏ Practical exercise ❏ Interactive class	❏ Beginner ❏ Intermediate ❏ Expert	❏ Orientation ❏ Annual ❏ Other _____	

_____ _____
Employee signature   *Observer signature*

Reference:
Perry, A. and Potter, P. 2006. *Clinical Nursing Skills & Techniques.* 6th ed. St. Louis, MO: Mosby Elsevier.

Evidence-Based Competency Management for the Medical-Surgical Unit, Second Edition

MS—Medical-Surgical

Name: _____ Date: _____

Skill: Pyxis Access

Steps	Completed	Comments
1. Signs on to Pyxis unit with ID number and code, then selects "remove med."		
2. Selects name of patient (if name does not appear, selects "enter ID" and types patient's last and first names and patient number). Presses enter to complete.		
3. Selects needed medication and quantity needed for the dose to be given. Presses enter.		
4. Removes only the requested amount.		
5. Closes the medication drawer completely then selects "quit" to complete transaction.		

Self-assessment	Evaluation/ validation methods	Levels	Type of validation	Comments
❏ Experienced ❏ Need practice ❏ Never done ❏ Not applicable (based on scope of practice)	❏ Verbal ❏ Demonstration/ observation ❏ Practical exercise ❏ Interactive class	❏ Beginner ❏ Intermediate ❏ Expert	❏ Orientation ❏ Annual ❏ Other _____	

_____   _____
Employee signature   *Observer signature*

Reference:
Duell, D., Martin, B., and Smith, S. 2008. *Clinical Nursing Skills: Basic to Advanced Skills*. 7th ed. Upper Saddle River, NJ: Pearson Education, Inc.

MS—Medical-Surgical

Name: _____ Date: _____

Skill: **Radial Artery Assessment**

Steps	Completed	Comments
1. Check the physician order. Explain the procedure to the patient. Obtain a complete history.		
2. Use the PVR machine and choose Upper Extremity Mode. Enter patient demographics and symptoms or indication for test.		
3. Under the VPR mode, obtain bilateral wrist waveforms.		
4. Using the Palmar Arch mode, obtain resting PPG Measurement of the first digit and record. Compress the radial artery and record. Proceed with all 10 digits.		
5. Place a copy of the report on the chart. Complete the file and enter into Datacheck.		

Self-assessment	Evaluation/ validation methods	Levels	Type of validation	Comments
❑ Experienced ❑ Need practice ❑ Never done ❑ Not applicable (based on scope of practice)	❑ Verbal ❑ Demonstration/ observation ❑ Practical exercise ❑ Interactive class	❑ Beginner ❑ Intermediate ❑ Expert	❑ Orientation ❑ Annual ❑ Other _____	

_____ _____
Employee signature   *Observer signature*

Reference:
Intersocietal Commission for the Accreditation of Vascular Laboratories, Society of Vascular Ultrasound, Society of Diagnostic Medical Sonography, and American Registry of Diagnostic Medical Sonography.

Evidence-Based Competency Management for the Medical-Surgical Unit, Second Edition

MS—Medical-Surgical

Name: _____ Date: _____

Skill: Rehab Unit Transfer Techniques

Steps	Completed	Comments
1. Evaluates the patient's physical and cognitive ability. (Reviews the chart, asks the patient to move his/her legs, squeezes hand, looks to the right, etc. Asks the patient questions that indicate his or her ability to understand what is being said.)		
2. Plans ahead. • Decides what to do, how to do it; gathers the necessary equipment and assistance.		
3. Adjusts the height of the bed according to the activity that will be completed with the patient. Lowers the side rail.		
4. Locks/secures the bed, wheelchair, cart, etc.		
5. Explains to the patient exactly what will be done and what he or she needs to do to help him or her self. Is specific and simple with instructions.		
6. Keeps the patient's body close during all transfers.		
7. Tightens abdominal muscles and locks upper body posture.		
8. Pivots feet, keeping at least on foot pointed in the direction of the patient as he or she lifts or moves his or her body.		
9. Lifts with legs, not back or arms.		
10. Lifts smoothly. When another staff member is assisting with the lift, uses a count such as "1, 2, 3, lift" to provide unity of movement.		
11. Knows physical limits and gets assistance when needed.		

Self-assessment	Evaluation/ validation methods	Levels	Type of validation	Comments
❏ Experienced ❏ Need practice ❏ Never done ❏ Not applicable (based on scope of practice)	❏ Verbal ❏ Demonstration/ observation ❏ Practical exercise ❏ Interactive class	❏ Beginner ❏ Intermediate ❏ Expert	❏ Orientation ❏ Annual ❏ Other _____	

_____ _____
Employee signature   *Observer signature*

Reference:
American Physical Therapy Association. 2007. *Standards of Practice for Physical Therapy*. Alexandria, VA: American Physical Therapy Association.

MS—Medical-Surgical

Name: _____ Date: _____

Skill: **Restraints (Role of Nursing Assistant)**

Steps	Completed	Comments
1. Verbalizes nursing assistant's role in safety evaluation of restraints.		
2. States how and where to document restraints.		
3. Soft restraints:		
a. Demonstrates how to remove and reapply soft restraint to extremity.		
b. Demonstrates how to secure to bed spring frame (not side rails) using slipknot.		
4. Mitt restraints:		
a. Demonstrates how to remove and reapply unit restraint.		
5. Leather restraints (optional):		
a. Demonstrates how to remove and reapply leather restraints.		
6. Verbalizes comprehension and support of nursing two-hour assessment of patient's restraints.		

Self-assessment	Evaluation/ validation methods	Levels	Type of validation	Comments
❏ Experienced ❏ Need practice ❏ Never done ❏ Not applicable (based on scope of practice)	❏ Verbal ❏ Demonstration/ observation ❏ Practical exercise ❏ Interactive class	❏ Beginner ❏ Intermediate ❏ Expert	❏ Orientation ❏ Annual ❏ Other _____	

_____   _____
Employee signature   *Observer signature*

Reference:
Perry, A. and Potter, P. 2006. *Clinical Nursing Skills & Techniques.* 6th ed. St. Louis, MO: Mosby Elsevier.

Name: _____ Date: _____

Skill: **Seclusion Restraint (Behavioral Health)**

Steps	Completed	Comments
Initiation of seclusion 1. Team of three or more staff and RN leader formed using principles of nonviolent crisis intervention.		
2. Leader informs patient of reason for restraints/seclusion and behaviors that must be exhibited to be released from seclusion.		
3. Leader directs team members and communicates with patient.		
4. When in room, patient searched, street clothes and dangerous objects removed, and patient placed in hospital gown.		
5. Vital signs obtained and documented. If unable to obtain vital signs due to patient's condition, documentation states reason for failure to obtain vital signs.		
6. Patient placed on mattress in seclusion room.		
7. Staff exit room one at a time.		
8. After patient secluded, staff critiques process (postvention).		
Documentation on seclusion/restraint log and orders 1. Documents patient's behavior leading to necessity of restraint/seclusion.		
2. Documents less restrictive means/alternatives to restraint/seclusion tried prior to seclusion.		
3. Discusses need for restraint/seclusion with patient/family and documents.		
4. Obtains physician order with clinical justification for restraints/seclusion within one hour of implementation of seclusion.		
5. Written order time-limited and does not exceed four hours.		
6. Initiates TV and audio monitoring and patient informed.		

MS—Medical-Surgical

7. Documents patient assessment and has signed by RN q 2h to determine if seclusion can be discontinued.		
8. Assesses patient's mental status and physical needs q 15 minutes and documented in log.		

Self-assessment	Evaluation/ validation methods	Levels	Type of validation	Comments
❑ Experienced ❑ Need practice ❑ Never done ❑ Not applicable (based on scope of practice)	❑ Verbal ❑ Demonstration/ observation ❑ Practical exercise ❑ Interactive class	❑ Beginner ❑ Intermediate ❑ Expert	❑ Orientation ❑ Annual ❑ Other _____	

_____   _____
Employee signature   *Observer signature*

Reference:
Joint Commission Resources. 2007. *Comprehensive Accreditation Manual for Hospitals: The Official Handbook.* Chicago, IL: The Joint Commission.

MS—Medical-Surgical

Name: _____ Date: _____

Skill: **Skin Burn, Care of**

Steps	Completed	Comments
1. Notifies physician of burn.		
2. Obtains physician order for:		
a. Sodium thiosulfate 5% sterile solution		
b. Cream/ointment for treatment		
3. Obtains sterile solution from pharmacy.		
4. Using a sterile gauze, applies solution to burned area.		
5. Rinses area with sterile water.		
6. Treats burned area as directed by physician utilizing ointment/cream.		

Self-assessment	Evaluation/ validation methods	Levels	Type of validation	Comments
❏ Experienced ❏ Need practice ❏ Never done ❏ Not applicable (based on scope of practice)	❏ Verbal ❏ Demonstration/ observation ❏ Practical exercise ❏ Interactive class	❏ Beginner ❏ Intermediate ❏ Expert	❏ Orientation ❏ Annual ❏ Other _____	

_____ _____
Employee signature *Observer signature*

Reference:
Perry, A. and Potter, P. 2006. *Clinical Nursing Skills & Techniques.* 6th ed. St. Louis, MO: Mosby Elsevier.

Evidence-Based Competency Management for the Medical-Surgical Unit, Second Edition

MS—Medical-Surgical

Name: _____ Date: _____

Skill: **Skin Prep Using Tincture of Iodine**

Steps	Completed	Comments
1. Screens patient for iodine allergy.		
2. Applies a thin layer of iodine/alcohol spray on skin prep area.		
3. Allows iodine/alcohol spray to completely dry.		
4. Asptically wipes excess spray.		
5. Checks for drips and pooled areas of spray.		
6. Covers/drapes prepped skin area.		

Self-assessment	Evaluation/ validation methods	Levels	Type of validation	Comments
❑ Experienced ❑ Need practice ❑ Never done ❑ Not applicable (based on scope of practice)	❑ Verbal ❑ Demonstration/ observation ❑ Practical exercise ❑ Interactive class	❑ Beginner ❑ Intermediate ❑ Expert	❑ Orientation ❑ Annual ❑ Other _____	

_____   _____

Employee signature   *Observer signature*

Reference:
Perry, A. and Potter, P. 2006. *Clinical Nursing Skills & Techniques.* 6th ed. St. Louis, MO: Mosby Elsevier.

MS—Medical-Surgical

Name: _____ Date: _____

Skill: **Staple/Clip Removal**

Steps	Completed	Comments
1. Verifies physician order for staple/clip removal.		
2. Identifies patient and explains procedure.		
3. Positions patient in a reclining position so that staples/clip are accessible and without undue tension.		
4. With povidone iodine or alcohol swab stick, begins cleansing incision line — midline, then each side — extending outward for an area of approximately 2." Uses a new stick for each stroke.		
5. Slides the lower jaws of the staple remover under the staple/clip to lift it.		
6. Squeezes (close) the handles of the remover, loosening the staple/clip.		
7. Gently lifts the staple/clip straight up and out of the skin.		
8. Continues to remove alternate staple/clip (third, fifth, etc.), assessing the wound for signs of dehiscence as each staple/clip is removed.		
9. Cleanses wound with povidone iodine or alcohol swab stick.		
10. Applies steristrips to wound if indicated.		
11. Documents procedure on patient's chart.		

Self-assessment	Evaluation/ validation methods	Levels	Type of validation	Comments
❏ Experienced ❏ Need practice ❏ Never done ❏ Not applicable (based on scope of practice)	❏ Verbal ❏ Demonstration/ observation ❏ Practical exercise ❏ Interactive class	❏ Beginner ❏ Intermediate ❏ Expert	❏ Orientation ❏ Annual ❏ Other _____	

_____   _____
Employee signature   *Observer signature*

Reference:
Perry, A. and Potter, P. 2006. *Clinical Nursing Skills & Techniques.* 6th ed. St. Louis, MO: Mosby Elsevier.

Evidence-Based Competency Management for the Medical-Surgical Unit, Second Edition

MS—Medical-Surgical

Name: _____ Date: _____

Skill: **Sterile Gloves, Applying**

Steps	Completed	Comments
1. Washes hands.		
2. Demonstrates opening package, protecting glove sterility.		
3. Applies glove #1 properly.		
4. Applies glove #2 properly.		
5. Removes gloves, protecting contamination of cleansed hands.		
6. Discusses concepts of working with a sterile field:		
a. Edges of field		
b. Glove contamination		

Self-assessment	Evaluation/ validation methods	Levels	Type of validation	Comments
❏ Experienced ❏ Need practice ❏ Never done ❏ Not applicable (based on scope of practice)	❏ Verbal ❏ Demonstration/ observation ❏ Practical exercise ❏ Interactive class	❏ Beginner ❏ Intermediate ❏ Expert	❏ Orientation ❏ Annual ❏ Other _____	

_____ _____
Employee signature *Observer signature*

Reference:
Duell, D., Martin, B., and Smith, S. 2008. *Clinical Nursing Skills: Basic to Advanced Skills*. 7th ed. Upper Saddle River, NJ: Pearson Education, Inc.

Name: _____ Date: _____

Skill: **Sterile Technique**

Steps	Completed	Comments
1. Dons sterile gloves without compromising sterility.		
2. Verbalizes process for assuring sterility of item/material has not been compromised:		
a. Seal		
b. Expiration date		

c. Appearance of
      • Container
      • Material		

3. Verbally defines boundaries of a sterile field.		
4. Demonstrates the following without compromising sterility/sterile field:		

a. Opens
      • Bottle/ampule
      • Package (e.g., syringe)
      • Tray/pack		

b. Passes sterile item from nonsterile person to sterile person/field:
      • Tech to nurse/physician
      • Tech to sterile receptacle		

c. Pours sterile fluid/material into sterile container/receptacle in sterile field.		

Self-assessment	Evaluation/validation methods	Levels	Type of validation	Comments
❏ Experienced ❏ Need practice ❏ Never done ❏ Not applicable (based on scope of practice)	❏ Verbal ❏ Demonstration/observation ❏ Practical exercise ❏ Interactive class	❏ Beginner ❏ Intermediate ❏ Expert	❏ Orientation ❏ Annual ❏ Other _____	

Employee signature

Observer signature

Reference:
Duell, D., Martin, B., and Smith, S. 2008. *Clinical Nursing Skills: Basic to Advanced Skills*. 7th ed. Upper Saddle River, NJ: Pearson Education, Inc.

MS—Medical-Surgical

Name: _____ Date: _____

Skill: Subcutaneous Needle Placement

Steps	Completed	Comments
1. Assembles equipment: BD Saf-T-Intima		
2. Identifies patient.		
3. Washes hands, wear gloves.		
4. Explains procedure.		
5. Selects appropriate insertion site. The sites that are most appropriate and most commonly used for SQ, they are upper arm, thigh, abdomen and upper chest.		
6. Primes tubing and needle – a. Remove control plug and prime. b. Replace control plug with PRN adapter.		
7. Release catheter sea by securing wing with fingers and pushing upward on segment below wing. Check level orientation.		
8. Cleanses site with Chloroprep swab.		
9. Insertion: a. Grip textured side of wings, pinch firmly. b. Pinch skin site between the thumb and forefinger of nondominant hand. c. Insert needle at 45 angle into skin fold up to hub of needle. d. Apply pressure to each wing. e. Grasp textured end of shield activator and withdraw needle stylet. f. Remove entire wire unit and discard in sharps.		
10. Connect tubing to PRN adapter.		
11. Secure wings with tape using H method.		
12. Places a semipermeable transparent dressing over site.		
13. States when to change site.		
14. Documents procedure.		

MS—Medical-Surgical

Self-assessment	Evaluation/ validation methods	Levels	Type of validation	Comments
❏ Experienced ❏ Need practice ❏ Never done ❏ Not applicable (based on scope of practice)	❏ Verbal ❏ Demonstration/ observation ❏ Practical exercise ❏ Interactive class	❏ Beginner ❏ Intermediate ❏ Expert	❏ Orientation ❏ Annual ❏ Other _____	

_____ _____
Employee signature   *Observer signature*

Reference:
Castaldi, P. 2005. *Clinical Nursing Skills and Techniques.* 6th ed. St. Louis, MO: Elsevier Mosby.

MS—Medical-Surgical

Name: _____ Date: _____

Skill: Tenckhoff Catheter

Steps	Completed	Comments
1. Gathers equipment: (2) Exam gloves (3) Betadine swab sticks (2) Sterile 4x4's (2) Sterile fenestrated gauze squares tape		
2. Utilizes body substance isolation; wash hands/wear gloves & mask on patient and nurse.		
3. Explain procedure to the patient.		
4. Remove dressing. Loosen tape and remove outer dressing. Put on gloves to remove remainder of dressing.		
5. Cleanse site. Using Chloroprep swab sticks, gently cleanse exit site starting at catheter and working outward in a circular pattern approximately 4 inches in diameters. Hydrogen peroxide may be used if patient is sensitive or has heavy crust formation. Dry with sterile 4x4's, starting at exit site and working outward in a circular pattern.		
6. Assess exit site for: bleeding, scab formation, crust formation, cuff extrusion, dialysis leakage, or purulent drainage.		
7. Signs of exit or tunnel infection: erythema, induration, exudates, unusual tenderness or pain or exuberant granulation or proud flesh. Report untoward symptoms to the physician.		

8. Dressing:
   1. Apply fenestrated gauze around catheter.
   2. Tape catheter to dressing in a curled fashion so that the catheter can be completely covered by additional gauze pads.
   3. Tape dressing in place, stabilizing catheter and tubing with tape bridges.
   4. Label with date, time and initials.
   5. Special dressing considerations:
      a. Avoid powders and ointments.
      b. Use the least amount of tape possible.
      c. Use hypoallergenic tape.
      d. Keep dressing free of moisture at all times.		

9. Documents in appropriate form.		

Self-assessment	Evaluation/ validation methods	Levels	Type of validation	Comments
❏ Experienced ❏ Need practice ❏ Never done ❏ Not applicable (based on scope of practice)	❏ Verbal ❏ Demonstration/ observation ❏ Practical exercise ❏ Interactive class	❏ Beginner ❏ Intermediate ❏ Expert	❏ Orientation ❏ Annual ❏ Other _____	

Employee signature

Observer signature

Reference:
Oncology Nursing Society. 2004. *Access Device Guidelines*. Philadelphia, PA: Oncology Nursing Society.

MS—Medical-Surgical

Name: _____ Date: _____

Skill: **Tissue Therapy**

Steps	Completed	Comments
1. Completes Braden Score on Admission Assessment.		
2. Implements nursing actions for Actual/Potential Impairment of Skin Integrity.		
3. Identifies stages of wounds. • Stage 1		
• Stage 2		
• Stage 3		
• Stage 4		
4. Describes interventions implemented for each wound stage. • Stage 1		
• Stage 2		
• Stage 3		
• Stage 4		
5. Verbalized how to use skin care products. • Stage 1		
• Stage 2		
• Stage 3		
• Stage 4		
6. Document on progress record.		

Self-assessment	Evaluation/ validation methods	Levels	Type of validation	Comments
❏ Experienced ❏ Need practice ❏ Never done ❏ Not applicable (based on scope of practice)	❏ Verbal ❏ Demonstration/ observation ❏ Practical exercise ❏ Interactive class	❏ Beginner ❏ Intermediate ❏ Expert	❏ Orientation ❏ Annual ❏ Other _____	

_____ _____
Employee signature   *Observer signature*

Reference:
Berstrom, et al. 1994. *Treatment of Pressure Ulcers*. U.S. Department of Health and Human Service.

Black, et al. 2007. National Pressure Ulcer Advisory Panel's Updated Ulcer Staging System. *Urology Nursing* 27(2): 144-150.

Name: _____ Date: _____

Skill: Tracheal Suctioning

Steps	Completed	Comments
A. Open suction system		
1. Elevates and extends patient's head, if possible.		
2. Opens suction kit and bottle of N/S.		
3. Carefully grasps cardboard edge of N/S tray and removes it from the suction kit.		
4. Pours N/S into tray.		
5. Preoxygentates patient by: a. Having patient take several deep breaths b. Manual use of BVM resuscitator with 100 % O^2 c. Pressing "sigh/100% O^2 suction" function pad on ventilator.		
6. If appropriate, loosens the ET tube and oxygen source connection at this time to allow easier, one-handed removal of the connection later.		
7. Puts on sterile gloves and removes catheter from kit.		
8. Approximates insertion depth from ostomy or end of ET tube to xiphoid process.		
9. Attaches catheter to suction source (hand touching suction tubing is no longer sterile).		
10. Tests patency of system and level of suction (80–120 mmHg) by occluding thumb air port and placing catheter tip in NS (NS will also lubricate catheter).		
11. Removes oxygen source.		
12. Without any suction applied, gently inserts the catheter until: a. Patient coughs b. Resistance is felt		
13. Applies suction and withdraws catheter in a rotating/twisting manner.		
14. Do not apply suction for more than 15 seconds at one time. The patient must be oxygenated between catheter passes made during a series of suctioning and at the end of the procedure.		

15. Flushes catheter and suction tubing with NS when the series is completed.		

16. Discards catheter and gloves by:
  a. Winding catheter around dominant hand and removing glove over catheter.
  b. Then, places gloved catheter in nondominant hand and removes the second glove over the gloved catheter.		

17. Applies oxygen source to patient, if applicable.		
18. Reassesses airway.		
B. Closed suction system		
1. Puts on clean gloves and sets suction high/full 150 mmHg or more.		
2. Connects catheter to suction tubing (if not already done). Note for tracheostomies: connects T-piece of short catheter to trach if not already in place; short catheter may be clipped to patient's gown between series of suctioning, if desired. Saves cap from suction connection for recapping when suction tubing is removed from catheter.		
3. Attaches 15 mL pop-top normal saline vial to irrigation port.		
4. Unlocks control valve.		
5. Observes the "black mark" on the catheter. The mark should be seen directly in front of the control valve when the catheter is completely withdrawn from the patient's airway.		

6. If a toilette/lavage is needed:
  a. Stabilizes the catheter T-piece and advances the catheter 4–5 inches (two short pushes).
  b. Gently pulsates the normal saline vial two to three times and allows the NS to flow down the outside of the catheter. Pulsating the vial gives better flow control to the NS.		

7. Gently advances catheter until patient coughs or resistance is felt. Does not remove oxygen source. Does not apply suction during insertion.		

8. Grasps control valve by placing open hand below valve. Places thumb across (perpendicular) lock-unlock mechanism. Presses down with thumb to apply suction.		
9. Slowly withdraws catheter (5–10 seconds) until the back mark is visible in front of the control valve.		
10. Pulsates NS vial to flush catheter between each pass of the catheter. When suctioning is completed, uses all the remaining NS to flush catheter. Removes vial and closes port.		
11. Locks the control valve.		
12. Turns off suction source.		
13. Leaves suction tubing connected, if desired.		
14. Reassesses patient.		
C. Documents procedure		

Self-assessment	Evaluation/ validation methods	Levels	Type of validation	Comments
❏ Experienced ❏ Need practice ❏ Never done ❏ Not applicable (based on scope of practice)	❏ Verbal ❏ Demonstration/ observation ❏ Practical exercise ❏ Interactive class	❏ Beginner ❏ Intermediate ❏ Expert	❏ Orientation ❏ Annual ❏ Other _____	

_____   _____

Employee signature   *Observer signature*

Reference:
Duell, D., Martin, B., and Smith, S. 2008. *Clinical Nursing Skills: Basic to Advanced Skills*. 7th ed. Upper Saddle River, NJ: Pearson Education, Inc.

MS—Medical-Surgical

Name: _____ Date: _____

Skill: Tracheostomy Care

Steps	Completed	Comments
1. Follows barrier precautions.		
2. Maintains sterile technique throughout procedure.		
3. Suctions trach secretions.		
4. Removes inner cannula and disposes of it.		
5. Removes soiled tracheostomy dressing.		
6. Sets up sterile field.		
7. Cleans skin area around trach with moistened H_2O_2.		
8. Inserts new sterile disposable inner cannula securely.		
9. Applies sterile tracheostomy dressing.		
10. Changes trach tape before removing soiled tape or uses disposable trach holder.		
11. Removes soiled trach tape with suture removal set scissors or disposable trach holder.		
12. Documents on Kardex as intervention.		

Self-assessment	Evaluation/ validation methods	Levels	Type of validation	Comments
❏ Experienced ❏ Need practice ❏ Never done ❏ Not applicable (based on scope of practice)	❏ Verbal ❏ Demonstration/ observation ❏ Practical exercise ❏ Interactive class	❏ Beginner ❏ Intermediate ❏ Expert	❏ Orientation ❏ Annual ❏ Other _____	

_____   _____
Employee signature   *Observer signature*

Reference:
Perry, A. and Potter, P. 2006. *Clinical Nursing Skills & Techniques*. 6th ed. St. Louis, MO: Mosby Elsevier.

Name: _____ Date: _____

Skill: Tracheostomy Tube Dislodgement, Emergency Intervention

Steps	Completed	Comments
1. Places the following equipment at bedside of all trach patients on admission to unit: a. Extra trach tube of same size as current trach. b. Trach tube with obturator one size smaller than current trach. c. Sterile hemostat or Kelly clamp. d. Hand held resuscitation device (AMBU Bag). e. Sterile gloves.		
2. Documents above bedside equipment on Kardex under Interventions; to be checked off each shift.		
3. In the event of an emergent trach dislodgement: a. Call for help. b. Position patient supine with head & neck extended. c. With sterile gloves & hemostats, spread open the trach stoma. d. Hold stoma open & administer O^2 until MD arrives. e. If patient on vent & has patent upper & lower airway, place occlusive dressing over stoma & ventilate with AMBU bag. If patient does not have patent upper & lower airway, ventilate through stoma. f. Assist MD with reinsertion of trach. g. If new trach is used, tape the new obturator to the head of the bed.		
4. Documents on the Interdisciplinary Progress Notes: a. Date & time of emergency procedure. b. Stoma & skin condition. c. Patient's respiratory status. d. Complications & actions taken. e. Patient's tolerance of procedure.		

MS—Medical-Surgical

Self-assessment	Evaluation/ validation methods	Levels	Type of validation	Comments
❑ Experienced ❑ Need practice ❑ Never done ❑ Not applicable (based on scope of practice)	❑ Verbal ❑ Demonstration/ observation ❑ Practical exercise ❑ Interactive class	❑ Beginner ❑ Intermediate ❑ Expert	❑ Orientation ❑ Annual ❑ Other _____	

_____
Employee signature

_____
Observer signature

Reference:
Roman, M. 2005. Tracheostomy tubes. *MedSurg Nursing* 14(2): 143-145.

MS—Medical-Surgical

Name: _____   Date: _____

Skill: **Transfer of Patient with Cervical Surgery and Patient with Shoulder Surgery**

Steps	Completed	Comments
1. Nurse is able to demonstrate ability to get patient in and out of bed.		
A. Getting up, explains procedure.		
1. Places patient in sitting position in bed, head of the bed up, foot of the bed down.		
2. Brings patient legs to edge of bed.		
3. Patient pivots bottom, may use draw sheet to assist.		
4. Squares patient on the bed with feet flat on the floor.		
5. May use side rail to assist with standing.		
B. Getting back to bed, explains procedure.		
1. Keep head of the bed up, may put side rail down.		
2. Has patient sit on edge of bed.		
3. Scoots bottom back up against head of bed.		
4. Leg closest to bottom of the bed elevates on to the bed first.		
5. As patient turns to get aligned, puts the other leg up on the bed.		

Self-assessment	Evaluation/ validation methods	Levels	Type of validation	Comments
❏ Experienced ❏ Need practice ❏ Never done ❏ Not applicable (based on scope of practice)	❏ Verbal ❏ Demonstration/ observation ❏ Practical exercise ❏ Interactive class	❏ Beginner ❏ Intermediate ❏ Expert	❏ Orientation ❏ Annual ❏ Other _____	

_____   _____
Employee signature   *Observer signature*

Reference:
Duell, D., Martin, B., and Smith, S. 2008. *Clinical Nursing Skills: Basic to Advanced Skills.* 7th ed. Upper Saddle River, NJ: Pearson Education, Inc.

Evidence-Based Competency Management for the Medical-Surgical Unit, Second Edition

MS—Medical-Surgical

Name: _____ Date: _____

Skill: Transfer Patient with Lumbar Surgery

Steps	Completed	Comments
1. Nurse demonstrates the ability to logroll patient.		
a. Shoulder and hip line.		
b. Rolls from back to side or side to back in one motion.		
c. Explains breathing technique to avoid tensing muscles and distract from pain.		
2. Nurse explains to patient how to get OOB.		
a. Side-lying position, has patient drop legs off the bed as he or she pushes his or her torso away from the bed. (Makes sure the head and foot of the bed are flat.)		
b. Breathing techniques used to distract from pain and decrease strain on sore muscles.		
3. Nurse explains return to bed.		
a. Bed remains flat. Patient stands with back of legs against the bed and hip against HOB side of rail.		
b. Patient is to sit down on bed, hands should hit the bed as buttocks does.		
c. Tells patient to lay down on side, elbow down, shoulder down, and head down. As the head goes down, the legs come up on the bed.		
d. Checks patient alignment before having patient turn to his or her back, repositions if necessary, has patient logroll to his back.		
e. Aligns patient in bed and pulls him or her up in bed if necessary before covering him or her up and leaving the room.		

Self-assessment	Evaluation/ validation methods	Levels	Type of validation	Comments
❏ Experienced ❏ Need practice ❏ Never done ❏ Not applicable (based on scope of practice)	❏ Verbal ❏ Demonstration/ observation ❏ Practical exercise ❏ Interactive class	❏ Beginner ❏ Intermediate ❏ Expert	❏ Orientation ❏ Annual ❏ Other _____	

Employee signature

Observer signature

Reference:
Duell, D., Martin, B., and Smith, S. 2008. *Clinical Nursing Skills: Basic to Advanced Skills*. 7th ed. Upper Saddle River, NJ: Pearson Education, Inc.

MS—Medical-Surgical

Name: _____ Date: _____

Skill: **Transfer, Transport, Ambulation**

Steps	Completed	Comments
1. States the rules for good body mechanics.		
2. Demonstrates dangling a patient.		
3. Transfers a patient between • Chair/bed and bed/chair. • Bed/stretcher and stretcher/bed.		
4. States guidelines for transporting patient from one area to another by • Wheelchair. • Stretcher.		
5. Demonstrates use of gait belt.		
6. States guidelines for assisting patient to ambulate.		
7. States care of a falling patient.		
8. Describes verification process for transporter: • Assuring the oxygen is hooked up correctly by licensed person. • Assures tubing and machines connected to patient are connected properly by asking for nursing staff assistance.		
9. Lists transporter responsibilities: Reports to nurse when patient wearing a "High Risk – Falls" yellow armband or patient is on oxygen is arriving to any unit		

Self-assessment	Evaluation/ validation methods	Levels	Type of validation	Comments
❑ Experienced ❑ Need practice ❑ Never done ❑ Not applicable (based on scope of practice)	❑ Verbal ❑ Demonstration/ observation ❑ Practical exercise ❑ Interactive class	❑ Beginner ❑ Intermediate ❑ Expert	❑ Orientation ❑ Annual ❑ Other _____	

_____ _____
Employee signature   *Observer signature*

Reference:
Duell, D., Martin, B., and Smith, S. 2008. *Clinical Nursing Skills: Basic to Advanced Skills*. 7th ed. Upper Saddle River, NJ: Pearson Education, Inc.

MS—Medical-Surgical

Name: _____ Date: _____

Skill: **Transportation of Postcatheterization Patients**

Steps	Completed	Comments
1. Verifies with RN that patient is able to be transported (patient stable, report given).		
2. Applies safety belt prior to transporting.		
3. Verifies RN and room readiness with appropriate nursing unit.		
4. Demonstrates proper transferring technique (from cart to bed with a second person assisting).		
5. Rechecks affected catheter site, distal pulse, and sandbag placement (notifies floor RN if any changes).		
6. Verifies floor staff is aware of patient arrival.		

Self-assessment	Evaluation/ validation methods	Levels	Type of validation	Comments
❏ Experienced ❏ Need practice ❏ Never done ❏ Not applicable (based on scope of practice)	❏ Verbal ❏ Demonstration/ observation ❏ Practical exercise ❏ Interactive class	❏ Beginner ❏ Intermediate ❏ Expert	❏ Orientation ❏ Annual ❏ Other _____	

_____   _____
Employee signature   *Observer signature*

Reference:
Duell, D., Martin, B., and Smith, S. 2008. *Clinical Nursing Skills: Basic to Advanced Skills.* 7th ed. Upper Saddle River, NJ: Pearson Education, Inc.

Evidence-Based Competency Management for the Medical-Surgical Unit, Second Edition

MS—Medical-Surgical

Name: _____   Date: _____

Skill: Tuberculosis Skin Test

Steps	Completed	Comments
1. Identifies order for TB test.		
2. Assesses patient for contraindications.		
• Previous positive test		
• Pregnant or breastfeeding		
3. Washes hands. Uses appropriate PPE.		
4. Gathers equipment and medication: • T.B. syringe with 26g needle • 5 TU/0.1 mL Tuburculin PPD • Alcohol swabs • Cotton ball		
5. Cleanses dorsal surface of forearm with alcohol swab, allows it to dry.		
6. Prepares syringe with 0.1 mL of 5 TU/0.1 mL of tuberculin, purified protein derivative (PPD).		
7. With level up enters skin on dorsal forearm about 4" below the elbow. Makes a wheal of approx. 6–10 mm.		
8. Reads test in 48–72° later. Measures only induration. Measures horizontal and vertical axis.		
9. Two-step testing: After reading initial site, places a second PPD wheal in opposite arm.		
10. Reads in 48–72°.		
11. Documents:		
• Date and site (right or left arm)		
• Date read and size 0x0, if negative, horizontal, and vertical size of induration only if present		

Self-assessment	Evaluation/ validation methods	Levels	Type of validation	Comments
❏ Experienced ❏ Need practice ❏ Never done ❏ Not applicable (based on scope of practice)	❏ Verbal ❏ Demonstration/ observation ❏ Practical exercise ❏ Interactive class	❏ Beginner ❏ Intermediate ❏ Expert	❏ Orientation ❏ Annual ❏ Other _____	

_____   _____
Employee signature   *Observer signature*

Reference:
Centers for Disease Control and Prevention. 2003. *Mantoux Tuberculin Skin Testing Training Materials Kit.*

MS—Medical-Surgical

Name: _____ Date: _____

Skill: **Urinary Catheterization**

Steps	Completed	Comments
Prior to preparing for procedure: Checks physician's orders for type of catheter to use and reviews patient's allergies and conditions. Checks with RN if questions arise from information collected. Assembles equipment.		
1. Uses sterile technique while preparing equipment.		
2. Checks balloon intactness by inflation and deflation prior to insertion.		
3. Cleanses meatal area.		
4. Inserts lubricated catheter.		
5. Verifies placement by urine return.		
6. Advances catheter 1"–2" further.		
7. Inflates balloon.		
8. Attaches to drainage bag placed below level of bladder.		
9. Verbalizes maximum amount of urine to be withdrawn at one time.		
10. Verbalizes P&P for clamping catheter to prevent bladder spasms and notification of registered nurse.		
11. Documents catheter insertion and urine return on patient Kardex and fluid record.		

Self-assessment	Evaluation/ validation methods	Levels	Type of validation	Comments
❑ Experienced ❑ Need practice ❑ Never done ❑ Not applicable (based on scope of practice)	❑ Verbal ❑ Demonstration/ observation ❑ Practical exercise ❑ Interactive class	❑ Beginner ❑ Intermediate ❑ Expert	❑ Orientation ❑ Annual ❑ Other _____	

_____ _____
Employee signature   **Observer signature**

Reference:
Duell, D., Martin, B., and Smith, S. 2008. *Clinical Nursing Skills: Basic to Advanced Skills*. 7th ed. Upper Saddle River, NJ: Pearson Education, Inc.

MS—Medical-Surgical

Name: _____ Date: _____

Skill: VAC: Negative Pressure Wound Therapy

Steps	Completed	Comments
1. Obtain equipment.		
a. VACD Suction Canister/tubing's/connectors/wound drain/clamps		

b. Gloves
     - Exam
     - Sterile		

c. Measuring guide		
d. Sterile cotton tip applicator		
e. Scissors		
f. Red Biohazard Bag		
g. Normal Saline		
h. Toppers (4x4) roll gauze/nonadherent impregnated gauze/foam (V.A.C.)/Duoderm (see what is needed)		
i. 30cc syringe with needle (if ordered)		
j. Clear occlusive drape (V.A.C.) transparent film dressing		
k. Skin Prep or No Sting Prep		
2. Identify patient - Two identifiers		
3. Explain procedure.		
4. Provide for privacy.		
5. Wash hands, set up sterile field.		
6. Do baseline assessment and measure wound (use exam gloves) - Apply sterile gloves		
7. Versatile One – - **Dressing Application:** Versatile One		
a. Apply a layer of **nonadherent impregnated gauze** (Adaptic) to wound bed.		
b. Open sterile packed silicone wound **drain** (flat/round/channel) and shorten the drain go 1" shorter than the wound bed by cutting off the end.		

Evidence-Based Competency Management for the Medical-Surgical Unit, Second Edition

MS—Medical-Surgical

c. Place the **drain** on top of the **nonadherent gauze** or envelope the **drain in gauze** and place into the wound bed on top of the nonadherent gauze. (never place directly on wound bed).		
d. Loosely fill wound with normal saline moistened gauze **(including undermining and tunneling)**		
e. Cover with transparent film **dressing**. The **dressing** should extend at least 1" around wound edges. Life the **drain** slightly where it exits the wound and pinch the dressing underneath it. If necessary, reinforce with waterproof tape in order to achieve tight seal.		
f. Slide the distal end of the **drain** through both round openings in the **clamp**. Leave **clamp** open. Use this **clamp** to temporarily disconnect the patient from the pump when desired.		
g. **Connect** the **drain** to the **connective tubing** by inserting the small end of the **Christmas tree tubing** connector into the drain.		
h. **Verify** seal. A good seal the dressing will contract noticeably when suction is turned on. Leak hear air escaping from the dressing. Seal not achieved, patch **dressing** with pieces of **transparent dressing** or **waterproof tape**.		
8. Suction - Set suction as indicated by physician order - Checks for leaks by clamping inspecting for ballooning of dsg		
9. Dressing Application: The V.A.C.		
a. Select V.A.C. dressing size to fill the entire wound cavity.		
b. For deeper wounds, larger pieces of trimmed foam dressing should be used in the wound to "build up" the overall dressing to obtain better coverage. If multiple pieces are used write the number used with permanent marker on the clear drape so all pieces will be removed when dressings are changed.		

c. Open dressing kit to clean dry surface and cut the V.A.C. foam to fit the size and shape of the wound including tunnels and undermined areas. (See recommended guidelines for foam choice).		
d. Size and trim drape to cover foam dressing, plus a 3-5cm border of intact skin.		
e. Do not discard excess drape: you may need it later as a patch.		
f. For fragile skin cut the drape to a size large enough to cover the foam dressing and the skin barrier layer only.		
g. Gently place the foam into the wound cavity, covering the entire wound base and sides, tunneling and undermining.		
h. If tunneling is present, measure tunnel with a sterile cotton tip applicator. Cut white (soft) foam in order to allow easy removal and contact with other foam pieces. After 2-3 dressing changes, only feed the foam to 1 cm of the distal end of the tunnel to allow closure by the growth of granulation tissue.		
i. Apply tubing to foam in wound. Tubing can be laid on top of the foam, or placed inside the foam dressing. The tubing should be positioned away from bony prominences.		
j. For deeper wounds, regularly reposition tubing to minimize pressure on wound edges. Cushion skin under tubing with excess foam to help hold tubing away from skin.		
k. Cover the foam and 3-5 cm of surrounding healthy tissue with drape to ensure an occlusive seal. Lift the tubing and pinch 1-3 cm of drape together under the tubing to help hold the tubing away from skin, pad underneath tubing to prevent leaks.		
l. Use excess drape to patch leaks and secure borders as needed.		

MS—Medical-Surgical

10. Suction:
  - Set suction as ordered standard initial setting 125 mmHg
  - Whistling sound indicates leak		

Self-assessment	Evaluation/ validation methods	Levels	Type of validation	Comments
❏ Experienced ❏ Need practice ❏ Never done ❏ Not applicable (based on scope of practice)	❏ Verbal ❏ Demonstration/ observation ❏ Practical exercise ❏ Interactive class	❏ Beginner ❏ Intermediate ❏ Expert	❏ Orientation ❏ Annual ❏ Other _____	

_____   _____
Employee signature   *Observer signature*

Reference:
Duell, D., Martin, B., and Smith, S. 2008. *Clinical Nursing Skills: Basic to Advanced Skills.* 7th ed. Upper Saddle River, NJ: Pearson Education, Inc.

MS—Medical-Surgical

Name: _____ Date: _____

Skill: Vacuum Assisted Closure Device (VACD) for Negative Pressure Wound Therapy (NPWT)

Steps	Completed	Comments
1. State purpose of Negative Pressure Wound Therapy (NPWT) dressings using Vacuum Assisted Closure Device (VACD).		
2. State **indications** and **contraindications** for use of VACD for NPWT.		
3. State what needs to be on physician order before placement or reapplication of VACD for NPWT.		
4. State what to look at when assessing wound for VACD dressing.		
5. State how often to do wound assessment and measurements and how to assess and measure.		
6. Obtain necessary equipment for dressing change. See policy.		
7. State what will they say and do with patient before beginning procedure.		
8. State what you look at to select the dressing size needed to best fit the wound.		
9. Dressing Application: 1. Select V.A.C. dressing size to fill the entire wound cavity.		
2. For deeper wounds, larger pieces of trimmed foam dressing should be used in the wound to "build up" the overall dressing to obtain better coverage. If multiple pieces are used write the number used with permanent marker on the clear drape so all pieces will be removed when dressings are changed.		
3. Apply skin prep to intact dry peri-wound skin, let air dry.		
4. Open dressing kit to clean dry surface and cut the V.A.C. foam to fit the size and shape of the wound including tunnels and undermined areas. (See recommended guidelines for foam choice).		

Evidence-Based Competency Management for the Medical-Surgical Unit, Second Edition

MS—Medical-Surgical

5. Size and trim drape to cover foam dressing, plus a 305 cm border of intact skin.		
6. Do not discard excess drape; you may need it later as a patch.		
7. For fragile skin cut the drape to a size large enough to cover the foam dressing and the skin barrier layer only.		
8. Gently place the foam into the wound cavity, covering the entire wound base and sides, tunneling and undermining.		
9. If tunneling is present, measure tunnel with a sterile cotton tip applicator. Cut white (soft) foam in order to allow easy removal and contact with other foam pieces. After 2-3 dressing changes, only feed the foam to 1 cm of the distal end of the tunnel to allow closure by the growth of granulation tissue.		
10. Apply skin prep to intact peri-wound skin.		
11. Cover the foam and 3-5 cm of intact peri-wound skin with a drape to ensure a seal. **DO NOT** pull or stretch drape over foam.		
12. Drape may be cut into multiple pieces for easier handling.		
13. Use excess drape to patch leaks and secure borders as needed.		
14. Pinch drape in a central area of dressing and cut a 1-2 cm hole through the drape.		
15. Apply TRAC pad directly over the hole.		
Applying "THE V.A.C." **1. Settings:** a. Standard initial setting is 125mmHg-200mmHg, depending on amount and size of wound.		
b. The setting may be decreased for patient tolerance.		
c. Usually continuous therapy is ordered.		
d. A physician order should be obtained for changing therapy settings.		
e. Remove canister from the sterile packaging, push it into the V.A.C. unit until it clicks in place.		

f. Connect the dressing tubing to the canister tubing. Make sure the clamps are open.		
g. A whistling sound may indicate a leak. Check areas around tubing for source of leaks. It is sometimes helpful to listen for potential leaks with a stethoscope around the dressing and tubing edges.		
h. Place the V.A.C. unit on a level of surface or hang from the footboard. Press in green power button, select new patient and adjust the V.A.C. until settings per physician order.		
i. Press **THERAPY ON/OFF** button to activate negative pressure therapy.		
j. If the canister is not engaged properly, the V.A.C. alarm will sound. Recheck the canister.		
k. When the negative pressure is activated, the sponge dressing should slowly compress into the wound if the seal is adequate.		
Disconnection/Reconnection: 1. **To Disconnect:** a. Turn the unit off.		
b. Clamp both clamps on the tubing.		
c. Press the quick release connector to separate the dressing tubing from the canister tubing.		
d. Cover the ends of the tubing with clean gauze and secure tape.		
2. **To Reconnect:** a. Remove the gauze from the ends of the tubing.		
b. Connect the tubing.		
c. Unclamp the clamps.		
d. Press V.A.C. green power button ON.		
e. Press therapy ON.		
Monitoring V.A.C.: 1. **Device Dressing** a. Visually check V.A.C. dressing for adequate seal – if leak detected, patch with additional pieces of tape.		
b. Signs of negative pressure every 2 hours.		

c. "Therapy on."		
d. Clamps open.		
e. Unkinked tubing.		
f. Pump settings.		
g. Increased bleeding or bloody drainage.		
h. Ineffective negative pressure allows drainage to accumulate and promote wound infection. V.A.C. therapy should not be interrupted for more than 2 hours a day. If therapy is to be interrupted for more than 2 hours change to a wet to moist dressing.		
Canister Change 1. Turn therapy off.		
2. Follow Body Substance Precautions to move the canister.		
3. Tighten clamps on canister tubing and dressing tubing.		
4. Disconnect canister tubing from dressing tubing.		
5. Pull back release knob on V.A.C. unit while simultaneously pulling the canister from the slot.		
6. Dispose of canister in a red bag and then dispose of bag in biohazard waste area.		
7. The V.A.C. canister should be changed with every dressing change or when full. If there is a large amount of drainage and you are changing the canister frequently notify physician immediately. Mark drainage amount as "output" on I&O sheet.		
8. Replace new canister and turn therapy on.		
Multiple Wounds 1. For assistance with application of V.A.C. dressing for multiple wounds contact Wound Care Center/Inpatient Wound Care Clinician.		
2. "Y" connector Part #202521-1 is available to treat multiple wounds.		

3. Wounds in close proximity can be treated by "bridging." Bridging involves protecting skin between two wounds with a drape, or Tegaderm or Duoderm, and applying a piece of foam to connect the two sponges.		
Dressing Removal: 1. Medicate patient as needed for pain prior to start of dressing removal.		
2. Press THERAPY ON/OFF to deactivate therapy.		
3. Disrupt clean drape and irate with saline to gently remove.		
4. Gently stretch the drape horizontally and slowly pull up from skin. Do not peel. Slowly remove foam from wound, adding saline if it adheres.		
5. Discard dressing by placing it in a red biohazard bag and then dispose the bag in the biohazard collection area.		
6. Let saline sit for 15-30 minutes. Pour directly on the foam after the transparent film is removed.		
7. Replace with normal saline dressing twice a day until further orders.		
8. When patient's treatment is discontinued send V.A.C. machine to Central Processing and notify Purchasing Department.		

Self-assessment	Evaluation/ validation methods	Levels	Type of validation	Comments
❑ Experienced ❑ Need practice ❑ Never done ❑ Not applicable (based on scope of practice)	❑ Verbal ❑ Demonstration/ observation ❑ Practical exercise ❑ Interactive class	❑ Beginner ❑ Intermediate ❑ Expert	❑ Orientation ❑ Annual ❑ Other _____	

_____ _____
Employee signature *Observer signature*

Reference:
Duell, D., Martin, B., and Smith, S. 2008. *Clinical Nursing Skills: Basic to Advanced Skills.* 7th ed. Upper Saddle River, NJ: Pearson Education, Inc.

MS—Medical-Surgical

Name: _____ Date: _____

Skill: Venous Reflux Exam

Steps	Completed	Comments
1. Checks physician order for appropriate test. Explains the procedure to the patient. Documents the patient history including past history of DVT, venous insufficiency, vein stripping, and varicose veins.		
2. Places the patient in a reverse trendelenburg position. Performs a physical assessment noting ulcers, discoloration, swelling, and varicosities.		
3. Performs a complete venous duplex exam using transverse compressions and doppler evaluation.		
4. Assesses for reflux at the following sites: • CFV • Saphenofemoral junction • Proximal-mid-distal SFV • GSV upper thigh • Lower thigh • Popliteal • LSV junction		
5. Documentation should include: varicosities, perforators, and reflux in seconds (retrograde doppler flow: 0.5 secs).		
6. Enters into datacheck. Completes worksheet.		

Self-assessment	Evaluation/ validation methods	Levels	Type of validation	Comments
❑ Experienced ❑ Need practice ❑ Never done ❑ Not applicable (based on scope of practice)	❑ Verbal ❑ Demonstration/ observation ❑ Practical exercise ❑ Interactive class	❑ Beginner ❑ Intermediate ❑ Expert	❑ Orientation ❑ Annual ❑ Other _____	

_____ _____
Employee signature   *Observer signature*

Reference:
Intersocietal Commission for the Accreditation of Vascular Laboratories, Society of Vascular Ultrasound, Society of Diagnostic Medical Sonography, and American Registry of Diagnostic Medical Sonography.

Name: _____ Date: _____

Skill: Ventilator—Assessment of the Patient and Troubleshooting

Steps	Completed	Comments
Is the patient connected to the ventilator?		
Is the ventilator plugged into a red emergency outlet?		
Listen to the sounds coming from the patient and ventilator. • Can you hear an actual air leak? • Check inflation of trach cuff or ascertain if Respiratory care has done this. • Patient coughing. • Secretions or mucus in the airway. • Patient "fighting" the ventilator. • Accumulation of water in the patient circuit. • Is patient able to speak?		
Observe all connections. Are they connected tightly? • Observe for kinking in the ventilator circuit. • In-line temp probe dislodged or missing?		
Observe the ventilator settings. Are they set correctly?		
Observe patient's activity level? • Is the patient coughing? • Is the patient turning over? • Is the patient breathing rapidly? • Is the patient anxious? • Subjectively is the patient dyspnic? • Is patient biting tube?		
Observe trach site and dressing.		
Auscultate breath sounds • Does the patient need suctioned?		
Take the patient's pulse oximetry reading.		
Take the patient's vital signs.		
Document findings.		

MS—Medical-Surgical

Self-assessment	Evaluation/ validation methods	Levels	Type of validation	Comments
❑ Experienced ❑ Need practice ❑ Never done ❑ Not applicable (based on scope of practice)	❑ Verbal ❑ Demonstration/ observation ❑ Practical exercise ❑ Interactive class	❑ Beginner ❑ Intermediate ❑ Expert	❑ Orientation ❑ Annual ❑ Other _____	

_____   _____
Employee signature   *Observer signature*

Reference:
Carlson, K. and Weigand, D. 2005. *AACN Procedure Manual for Critical Care*. 5th ed. St. Louis, MO: Elsevier Saunders. 861-869.

MS—Medical-Surgical

Name: _____ Date: _____

Skill: **Vital Signs (Observation Room)**

Steps	Completed	Comments
1. Identifies patient and explains procedure.		
2. Demonstrates proper use of IVAC thermometer and notifies RN of temp greater than 99.5°.		
3. Observes heart rate. Notifies RN if HF is increased or decreased by 20 points from initial observation room reading (or notifies RN if HR is less than 60 or greater than 110).		
4. Correctly applies appropriate-sized blood pressure cuff and observes normal blood pressure reading.		
5. Identifies arterial blood pressure reading from monitor. Notifies RN if BP increases or decreases by 20 (or if systolic blood pressure increases above 160 or systolic blood pressure decreases below 100).		
6. Observes and counts respirations effectively and notifies RN if respiration rate is lower than 12 or greater than 24.		
7. Documents appropriate vital signs, in correct intervals, on observation room flowsheet.		

Self-assessment	Evaluation/ validation methods	Levels	Type of validation	Comments
❏ Experienced ❏ Need practice ❏ Never done ❏ Not applicable (based on scope of practice)	❏ Verbal ❏ Demonstration/ observation ❏ Practical exercise ❏ Interactive class	❏ Beginner ❏ Intermediate ❏ Expert	❏ Orientation ❏ Annual ❏ Other _____	

_____   _____
Employee signature   *Observer signature*

Reference:
Duell, D., Martin, B., and Smith, S. 2008. *Clinical Nursing Skills: Basic to Advanced Skills.* 7th ed. Upper Saddle River, NJ: Pearson Education, Inc.

Evidence-Based Competency Management for the Medical-Surgical Unit, Second Edition

MS—Medical-Surgical

Name: _____ Date: _____

Skill: Weights/Height

Steps	Completed	Comments
1. Selects appropriate scale, standing or bed scale.		
2. Identifies patient by checking name on ID band.		
3. Provide privacy and explain procedure to patient.		
Standing Scale:		
4. Have patient remove robe.		
5. Assist patient on scales and remains close to prevent falls.		
6. **For the digital scale:** turn on scale - be sure it is at 0.0. If not, hit the "zero" button on the left of the display. Weigh patient following the directions on the scale. **For balance weight scale:** Move both riders to the left and be sure the scale bar is balanced. Determine weight by sliding the rider into the grove closest to patient's estimated weight. Move the riders until the scale balances and add the sum of both.		

7. **Height:**
  a. While patient is standing, ask to stand straight with feet flat on scale.
  b. Raise the measuring rod above the patient's head.
  c. Lower the rod until it rests on the top of the patient's head.
  d. Note the patient's height in inches.
  e. Raise the measuring rod and fold down.
  f. Help the patient off scale if needed.		

8. Assist patient back to bed.		
9. Record weight and height.		
Bed Scale 10. Position scale next to bed and lock wheels. Then turn patient away from scale. Remove excess linen.		
11. Roll patient back onto scale stretcher. Raise stretcher off bed 2 inches.		

12. Determine weight.		
13. Lower patient onto mattress and remove scale stretcher from under patient.		
14. Leave patient in comfortable position.		
15. Record weight and the number/type scale used. Use the SAME scale for the SAME patient as much as possible.		
16. Return scale to proper storage area.		

Self-assessment	Evaluation/ validation methods	Levels	Type of validation	Comments
❏ Experienced ❏ Need practice ❏ Never done ❏ Not applicable (based on scope of practice)	❏ Verbal ❏ Demonstration/ observation ❏ Practical exercise ❏ Interactive class	❏ Beginner ❏ Intermediate ❏ Expert	❏ Orientation ❏ Annual ❏ Other _____	

_____ _____
Employee signature   *Observer signature*

Reference:
Perry, A. and Potter, P. 2006. *Clinical Nursing Skills & Techniques.* 6th ed. St. Louis, MO: Mosby Elsevier.

MS—Medical-Surgical

Name: _____ Date: _____

Skill: **Wound Cultures**

Steps	Completed	Comments
1. Checks the physician's order.		
2. Makes out the appropriate requisition. Makes out a label.		
3. Gathers equipment: culturette 11 or minitip gloves.		
4. Uses principles of BSI.		
Open wounds: 1. Uses culturette 11. Swabs area of most purulence in a rotating manner while avoiding contact with skin.		
Dry lesions: 1. Moistens culturette 11 swabs with sterile saline. Swabs lesions.		
2. Makes sure both swabs contain specimen. The first is used for gram smear, and the second is for culture.		

Sinus tracts:
 	
1. Cleanses orifice of tract with antiseptic solution:
   a. Uses minitip culturette.
   b. Using care not to touch skin, inserts minitip culturette.
   c. Advances swab using upward motion and rotates to obtain specimen (only physician may aspirate material).		

2. Places culturettes in containers and breaks ampule.		
3. Labels and bags all specimens and sends to lab as soon as possible. (Labels with area from which wound culture obtained.)		
4. Charts date and time wound culture obtained and sent to lab.		

Self-assessment	Evaluation/ validation methods	Levels	Type of validation	Comments
❏ Experienced ❏ Need practice ❏ Never done ❏ Not applicable (based on scope of practice)	❏ Verbal ❏ Demonstration/ observation ❏ Practical exercise ❏ Interactive class	❏ Beginner ❏ Intermediate ❏ Expert	❏ Orientation ❏ Annual ❏ Other _____	

_____

Employee signature

_____

Observer signature

Reference:
Duell, D., Martin, B., and Smith, S. 2008. *Clinical Nursing Skills: Basic to Advanced Skills.* 7th ed. Upper Saddle River, NJ: Pearson Education, Inc.

MS—Medical-Surgical

Name: _____ Date: _____

Skill: **Wound Photography**

Steps	Completed	Comments
1. Obtains appropriate equipment: • Camera(s) • Wound labels • "Blue pad" or other drape for background.		
2. Labels wound with Pt. ID#, initials, date, and wound #.		
3. Selects the appropriate magnifications for the size of the wound. Uses previous magnification. If new patient, documents magnification used.		
4. Multiple wounds: takes a reference photo of the limb/area at 1:5 or larger.		
5. Reviews procedure for photography of circumferential wounds (anterior, lateral, posterior, medial photos).		
6. Reviews procedure for processing via film mailer.		

Self-assessment	Evaluation/ validation methods	Levels	Type of validation	Comments
❏ Experienced ❏ Need practice ❏ Never done ❏ Not applicable (based on scope of practice)	❏ Verbal ❏ Demonstration/ observation ❏ Practical exercise ❏ Interactive class	❏ Beginner ❏ Intermediate ❏ Expert	❏ Orientation ❏ Annual ❏ Other _____	

_____   _____
Employee signature   *Observer signature*

Reference:
Berstrom, et al. 1994. *Treatment of Pressure Ulcers*. U.S. Department of Health and Human Services.

Name: _____ Date: _____

Skill: Zoladex, Subcutaneous Injection of

Steps	Completed	Comments
1. Washes hands.		
2. Gathers catheter equipment: Zoladex implant, alcohol swabs, 1 % lidocaine hydrochloride, 1 mL T.B. syringe, bandage.		
3. Positions patient in supine position and drapes to expose abdomen.		
4. Selects injection site in one of four abdominal quadrants at least 5 cm (2 in.) away from umbilicus. Makes sure site is free of rashes, bruises, or scars.		
5. Cleans area on upper abdominal wall with alcohol sponge.		
6. Draws up 0.2 to 0.5 mL of 1% lidocaine hydrochloride into TB syringe.		
7. Stretches skin at injection site with one hand.		
8. Holds T.B. syringe at 15° angle to skin and with bevel up.		
9. Inserts needle into dermis.		
10. Injects lidocaine to form a bleb.		
11. Inspects Zoladex syringe drug chamber for presence of drug.		
12. Inserts the needle with bevel up at 45° angle into subcutaneous fat at the site of the bleb.		
13. Does not aspirate. (If blood appears in syringe, withdraws and obtains new syringe.)		
14. Changes direction of needle so it is parallel to abdominal wall.		
15. Pushes needle in.		
16. Then withdraws about 1 cm.		
17. Depresses plunger.		
18. Withdraws needle and bandage site with Band-Aid.		
19. Inspects tip of needle to assure medication has been discharged.		

MS—Medical-Surgical

20. Discards both syringes into sharps container.		
21. Monitors site for bleeding or bruising.		
22. Educates patient: • What implant looks like • Possible bleeding • Reactions: hot flashes, decreased strength, gynocosmastia, sexual dysfunction		
23. Removes tear-off portion of package and affixes to patient's record.		
24. Documents injection.		

Self-assessment	Evaluation/ validation methods	Levels	Type of validation	Comments
❏ Experienced ❏ Need practice ❏ Never done ❏ Not applicable (based on scope of practice)	❏ Verbal ❏ Demonstration/ observation ❏ Practical exercise ❏ Interactive class	❏ Beginner ❏ Intermediate ❏ Expert	❏ Orientation ❏ Annual ❏ Other _____	

_____ _____

Employee signature *Observer signature*

Reference:
Cooley, C. and Morgan, G. 2005. Injection system for two luteinizing hormone-releasing hormone agonists: A comparative assessment of administration times and nurses' perceptions. *European Journal of Oncology Nursing* 9(4): 334-340.

ROLE

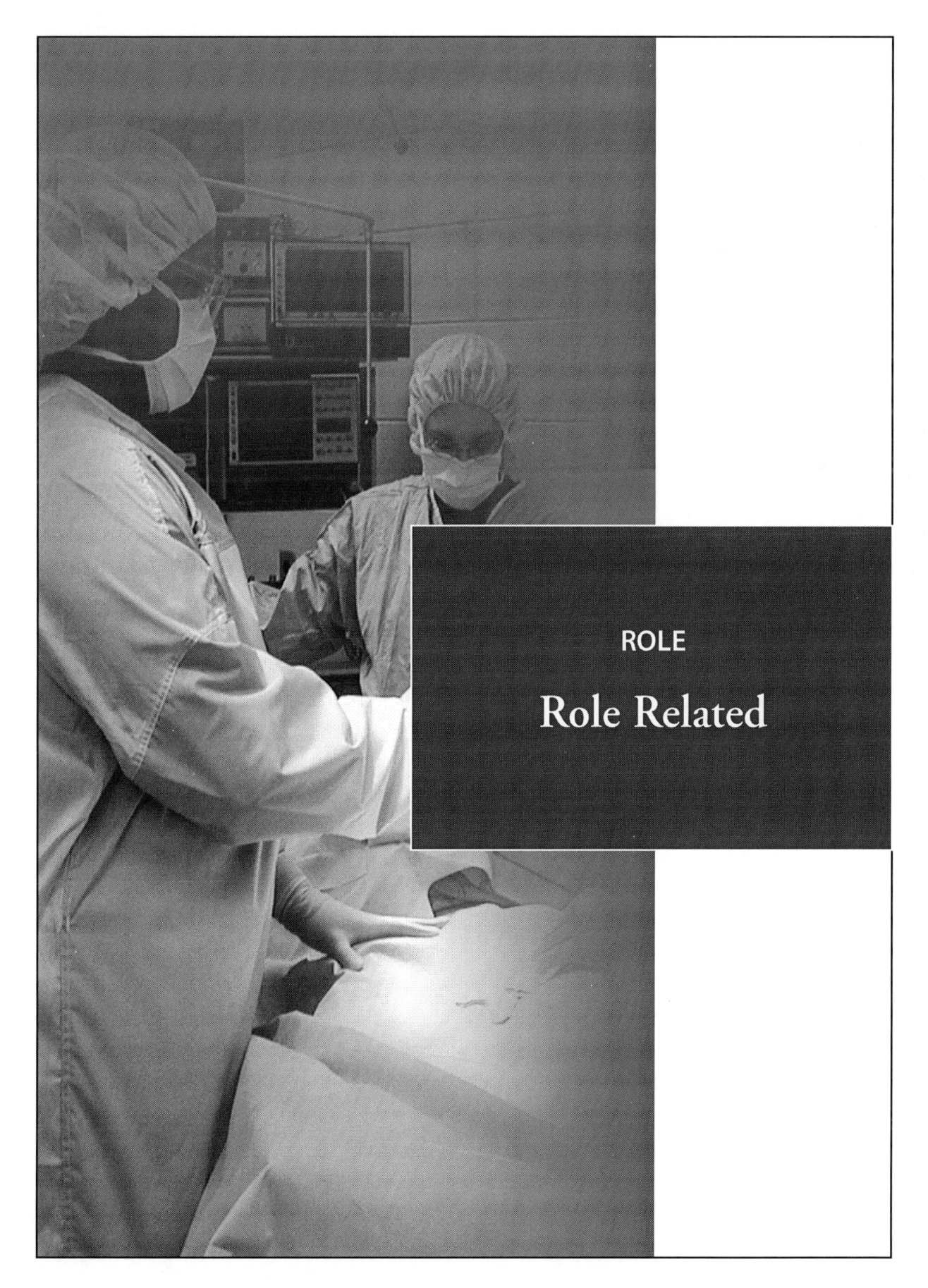

Role Related

ROLE—Role Related

Contents

Acid Mixing 317
Adding Toner to Fax 318
Administrative Associate Accurate Charging 319
Age-Specific Competency Checklist RN/LPN 320
Age-Specific Competency Checklist SA/AA 322
Appointment Scheduling—Diabetes Center 324
Behavioral Health Associate 325
Bicarb Mixing 326
Charge Entry 327
Charge Nurse Assessment/Evaluation 328
Defibrillator Function—Daily Check (Lifepak 9) 333
Discharge Bed/Bassinette Cleaning for Environmental Associates 334
HOP Charges 336
Insurance Precertification Authorization 337
LPN Skills Assessment/Evaluation 338
Nursing Assistant Orientation Skills Assessment/Evaluation 341
Nursing Student Technician Competency Checklist 346
Private Duty RN/LPN Competency Evaluation 348
Registration 349
RN Skills Assessment/Evaluation 350
Sitter Guidelines/Expectations 354
Telephone Skills 358
Telephone Skills (Problem Solving) 359
Unit Secretary Orientation Skills Assessment/Evaluation 360

ROLE—Role Related

Name: _____ Date: _____

Skill: Acid Mixing

Steps	Completed	Comments
1. Rinses tank (only if changing type of acid). Rinses tank: • Sprays inside of tank with hose. • Opens water valve (red valve on side of vat) and add some water. • Opens manual drain briefly. • Opens drain valve and turn on transfer pump to drain remaining fluid. • Turns off transfer pump.		
2. Obtains appropriate acid supply boxes (2 or 3k). Fills tank to 15–20 gallons and then adds liquid mix. Always add liquid first.		
3. Turns bicarb mixer 2 on and then adds dry powder: red, green, then white bags. Always in that order.		
4. Turns mixer off when tank gets close to two-gallon mark. Turns off water supply to tank when level reaches 25 gallons.		
5. Turns mixer back on and runs until it automatically shuts off (approximately 10 minutes).		
6. Is certain which acid was mixed (2k or 3k) and puts label on vat.		
7. Opens proper valve (2k or 3k). (All other valves should be closed.)		
8. Turns off transfer pump, watches level in the tank, and turns off transfer pump when tank is empty.		

Self-assessment	Evaluation/ validation methods	Levels	Type of validation	Comments
❑ Experienced ❑ Need practice ❑ Never done ❑ Not applicable (based on scope of practice)	❑ Verbal ❑ Demonstration/ observation ❑ Practical exercise ❑ Interactive class	❑ Beginner	❑ Orientation ❑ Annual ❑ Other _____	

_____   _____
Employee signature   **Observer signature**

Evidence-Based Competency Management for the Medical-Surgical Unit, Second Edition

ROLE—Role Related

Name: _____ Date: _____

Skill: Adding Toner to Fax

Steps	Completed	Comments
1. Watch for "add toner" light.		
2. Open cartridge cover by pulling the lever above the arrow mark.		
3. Remove the old cartridge.		
4. Remove a new cartridge from the protective bag.		
5. Rock the new cartridge five or six times to distribute the toner evenly inside the cartridge.		
6. Place the cartridge on a flat, clean surface.		
7. Steady the cartridge with one hand and remove the seal by gently pulling on the plastic tab with your other hand.		
8. Load the cartridge in the direction indicated by the arrow.		
9. Gently slide the cartridge into the printer until it is down inside the main unit and level.		
10. Close the cartridge cover.		

Self-assessment	Evaluation/ validation methods	Levels	Type of validation	Comments
❏ Experienced ❏ Need practice ❏ Never done ❏ Not applicable (based on scope of practice)	❏ Verbal ❏ Demonstration/ observation ❏ Practical exercise ❏ Interactive class	❏ Beginner ❏ Intermediate ❏ Expert	❏ Orientation ❏ Annual ❏ Other _____	

_____   _____

Employee signature   *Observer signature*

ROLE—Role Related

Name: _____ Date: _____

Skill: Administrative Associate Accurate Charging

Steps	Completed	Comments
1. Demonstrates accurate charging with the following items:		
a. Apnea management		
b. Exchange transfusion		
c. Resuscitation		
d. IV insertion		
e. Cascade set-up		
f. Vent set-up		
g. Survanta		
h. Disposable LP tray		
i. Pulse oximeter		
j. Pulse oximeter checks		
k. Neonatal transport (up to one and a half hours)		
l. Neonatal transport (additional half hour)		
m. Circumcision		
n. Cardiac respiratory monitors		
o. Apnea homecare training		
p. Phototherapy		
q. Eye exams		
r. Syringe pump (feeds)		
s. Syringe pump (meds)		
t. Disposable BP cuffs		
2. Batches items and sends to data processing.		

Self-assessment	Evaluation/ validation methods	Levels	Type of validation	Comments
❏ Experienced ❏ Need practice ❏ Never done ❏ Not applicable (based on scope of practice)	❏ Verbal ❏ Demonstration/ observation ❏ Practical exercise ❏ Interactive class	❏ Beginner ❏ Intermediate ❏ Expert	❏ Orientation ❏ Annual ❏ Other _____	

_____ _____
Employee signature   *Observer signature*

Evidence-Based Competency Management for the Medical-Surgical Unit, Second Edition

ROLE—Role Related

Name: _____ Date: _____

Skill: Age-Specific Competency Checklist RN/LPN

Steps	Completed	Comments
Alters care given on age-specific needs.		
A. Physical		
Adolescent – increases need for nourishment/nutrition.		
Early adulthood – alters diet, decreases amount of food.		
Middle adult – provides assistance with ambulation, provides moisture, keeps temperature set for comfort.		
Late adult – close observation of vital signs, I&O stays alert for drug-drug interactions.		
B. Motor/sensory adaptation		
Adolescent – assists with ambulation, provides for sleep.		
Early adulthood – ensures decreased background noise, encourages use of glasses.		
Middle adult – speaks loudly, assists with ambulation.		
Late adult – does not rush patient; provides glasses, hearing aids for assistance.		
C. Cognitive		
Adolescent – speaks to patient as an adult not a child.		
Early adulthood – identifies learning preferences.		
Middle adult – alters patient education techniques.		
Late adult – encourages participation in society, social groups.		
D. Psychosocial		
Adolescence – encourages peers to visit/phone, explores feelings with patients.		

Early adulthood – explores how illness will stress job, family, and responsibilities.		
Middle adult – helps patient identify stressors and his or her relationship to illness.		
Late adult – assesses patient's place in society, addresses concerns.		

Self-assessment	Evaluation/ validation methods	Levels	Type of validation	Comments
❏ Experienced ❏ Need practice ❏ Never done ❏ Not applicable (based on scope of practice)	❏ Verbal ❏ Demonstration/ observation ❏ Practical exercise ❏ Interactive class	❏ Beginner ❏ Intermediate ❏ Expert	❏ Orientation ❏ Annual ❏ Other _____	

_____   _____
Employee signature   *Observer signature*

ROLE—Role Related

Name: _____ Date: _____

Skill: Age-Specific Competency Checklist SA/AA

Steps	Completed	Comments
Alters care based on age-specific needs.		
A. Physical		
Adolescent – provides snacks.		
Early adulthood – provides alternative foods within diet.		
Middle adult – sets room temperature for patient comfort.		
Late adult – measures urine output, reports changes to nurse.		
B. Motor/sensory adaptation		
Adolescent – assists with ambulation, provides for rest.		
Early adulthood – keeps area quiet.		
Middle adult – speaks slowly, assists with ambulation.		
Late adult – does not rush patient.		
C. Cognitive		
Adolescent – treats patient as an adult.		
Early adulthood – helps patient to alleviate boredom.		
Middle adult – repeats instructions as needed—answers questions.		
Late adult – encourages activities.		
D. Psychosocial		
Adolescent – encourages patient to talk, participate.		
Early adulthood – participates in identification of stress of patient and reports to nurse.		

ROLE—Role Related

Middle adult – participates in identification of stressors and reports to nurse.		
Late adult – encourages participant in ADLs—offers to help when needed.		

Self-assessment	Evaluation/ validation methods	Levels	Type of validation	Comments
❏ Experienced ❏ Need practice ❏ Never done ❏ Not applicable (based on scope of practice)	❏ Verbal ❏ Demonstration/ observation ❏ Practical exercise ❏ Interactive class	❏ Beginner ❏ Intermediate ❏ Expert	❏ Orientation ❏ Annual ❏ Other _____	

_____   _____

Employee signature   *Observer signature*

ROLE—Role Related

Name: _____   Date: _____

Skill: Appointment Scheduling—Diabetes Center

Steps	Completed	Comments
1. Determines accurate spelling of patient's full name on outpatient order form.		
2. Contacts patient for scheduling within one business day after receiving the order.		
3. Notifies physician and diabetes center staff of scheduling problems with a patient.		
4. Schedules correct appointment type with appropriate information given to the patient regarding the appointment and what to bring.		
5. Documents patient's insurance information and refers patient to patient account services when appropriate.		
6. Instructs patient to call his or her insurance company to check on coverage for diabetes education prior to coming to the first appointment.		
7. Obtains approval from the educator for overbooking appointments, based on patient's needs.		

Self-assessment	Evaluation/ validation methods	Levels	Type of validation	Comments
❑ Experienced ❑ Need practice ❑ Never done ❑ Not applicable (based on scope of practice)	❑ Verbal ❑ Demonstration/ observation ❑ Practical exercise ❑ Interactive class	❑ Beginner ❑ Intermediate ❑ Expert	❑ Orientation ❑ Annual ❑ Other _____	

_____   _____
Employee signature   *Observer signature*

ROLE—Role Related

Name: _____ Date: _____

Skill: **Behavioral Health Associate**

Steps	Completed	Comments
A. Phlebotomy & Advanced Technical Skills:		
1. Veinpuncture procedure		
2. Finger stick procedure		
3. Blood bank procedure		
4. Quality Control procedure		
5. Blood Glucose Testing procedure		
6. Blood pressure		
B. Review: Demonstrates ability to obtain and transport appropriately the following specimens:		
1. Sputum		
2. Urine/Routine/CCMS		
3. Stool		
4. Blood		

Self-assessment	Evaluation/ validation methods	Levels	Type of validation	Comments
❏ Experienced ❏ Need practice ❏ Never done ❏ Not applicable (based on scope of practice)	❏ Verbal ❏ Demonstration/ observation ❏ Practical exercise ❏ Interactive class	❏ Beginner ❏ Intermediate ❏ Expert	❏ Orientation ❏ Annual ❏ Other _____	

_____   _____
Employee signature   *Observer signature*

Evidence-Based Competency Management for the Medical-Surgical Unit, Second Edition

ROLE—Role Related

Name: _____ Date: _____

Skill: Bicarb Mixing

Steps	Completed	Comments
1. Checks that mix tank is empty and clean.		
2. Checks that valve 8D is closed.		
3. Determines batch size to be made, 50 to 100 gallons. (We average 150–200 gal. per day.)		
4. For 100 gal., turns fill to "on" and presses "fill start." When mix tank has filled to 95 gal., marks it (automatically shuts off). (Takes approx. 30 minutes.)		
5. For 50 gal, turns fill to "on" and presses "fill start." When mix tank reaches 45 gal., marks it, turns fill switch to "off."		
6. Opens valve 6M.		
7. Turns mix to "on" and presses "mix start." Add dry chemical to mix tank (one bag per 25 gal.). It will mix for 30 minutes and has auto shut-off.		
8. After mix is complete, checks that all dry chemical has dissolved.		

Self-assessment	Evaluation/ validation methods	Levels	Type of validation	Comments
❏ Experienced ❏ Need practice ❏ Never done ❏ Not applicable (based on scope of practice)	❏ Verbal ❏ Demonstration/ observation ❏ Practical exercise ❏ Interactive class	❏ Beginner ❏ Intermediate ❏ Expert	❏ Orientation ❏ Annual ❏ Other _____	

_____ _____
Employee signature   *Observer signature*

ROLE—Role Related

Name: _____ Date: _____

Skill: **Charge Entry**

Steps	Completed	Comments
1. User performs entering a charge from start to finish.		
2. Demonstrates changing the date and quality fields.		
3. Explains the ramifications of exiting out of the change screen without using the update button.		
4. Identifies when, why, and how to change an account before entering a charge.		

Self-assessment	Evaluation/ validation methods	Levels	Type of validation	Comments
❏ Experienced ❏ Need practice ❏ Never done ❏ Not applicable (based on scope of practice)	❏ Verbal ❏ Demonstration/ observation ❏ Practical exercise ❏ Interactive class	❏ Beginner ❏ Intermediate ❏ Expert	❏ Orientation ❏ Annual ❏ Other _____	

_____   _____
Employee signature   *Observer signature*

Evidence-Based Competency Management for the Medical-Surgical Unit, Second Edition

ROLE—Role Related

Name: _____ Date: _____

Skill: **Charge Nurse Assessment/Evaluation**

Steps	Completed	Comments
A. Clinical/Technical Competencies: *Responsibilities directly related to patient care or some technical aspect of working on a clinical unit.* 1. Enter patient acuities into Optilink computer (or ensure these are done) according to policy.		
2. Assist staff in completing their work.		
3. Act as a clinical resource, sharing knowledge.		
4. Use computer skills to chart and complete reports.		
5. Delegate workload appropriately and fairly.		
6. Check emergency equipment handle unit emergencies.		
7. Conducts initial unitwide patient assessments.		
8. Knowledge of medical equipment to provide care.		
9. Knowledgeable of available clinical resources when needed.		
10. Knowledgeable of unit, type of patients, procedures, etc. to plan work.		
11. Maintain a safe, clean physical unit environment.		
12. Provide direct care as needed, balancing patient care with charge nurse duties.		
13. Give an effective change of shift report to oncoming Charge Nurse.		
14. Coordinates shift assignments for all staff and delegates patient care according to patient acuity, assures nursing assistants will be given specific patient care assignments.		
15. Facilitates patient safety.		
B. Critical Thinking Competencies: *Responsibilities that address effective decision making and problem solving involving both critical and operational issues on the unit.* 1. Anticipate patient needs, staffing requirements; engage in anticipatory planning and generating solutions.		

2. Assess/evaluate clinical and operational information.		
3. Manage crises as they occur.		
4. Make decisions.		
5. Uses good judgment.		
6. Prioritizes—decides the order of importance of tasks.		
7. Uses knowledge of patient status to plan care.		
8. Uses knowledge of staff capabilities to plan care.		
9. Troubleshoot—problem solve to prevent a potential crisis.		
10. Manage time effectively.		
11. Assess requirements and takes action to provide adequate staff.		
12. Know and deal with personal limitations.		
13. Deal effectively with change.		
C. **Organizational Competencies:** *Responsibilities to understand and operate in the organizational environment on the unit as well as in the larger institutions (hospital, agency, etc.).* 1. Coordinate multiple tasks in order to keep unit operations flowing.		
2. Deal with interruptions.		
3. Uses a method to keep organized.		
4. Prepare prior to the beginning of shift.		
5. Know and use hospital/unit policies and patient procedures appropriately.		
6. Oversee unit functions to ensure overall quality of care/practice.		
7. Coordinate the following functions:		
a. TTO/Floating under the direction of the Unit Manager/Administrative Supervisor.		
b. The Float nurse's assignment. Acts as a resource to the float nurse.		
c. Relocated staff during emergencies.		
d. Assures completeness of staff partnership assignments sheet.		

ROLE—Role Related

8. Reviews staffing patterns for the oncoming shift with the Unit Manager. Assigns nursing assistants to the RN leaders/and partnerships. At shift change (i.e. 3:00pm) the Charge Nurse reviews the assignments for nursing assistants in collaboration with the partnership leaders. Together they determine what remaining tasks need to be completed and delegates these tasks to the oncoming nursing assistant to partnership as needed, in collaboration with the Charge Nurse that is leaving.		
9. Assigns breaks and lunches and marks on board/assignment sheet.		
a. Staff report on and off the unit to the Charge Nurse. The staff documents and/or verbally reports the time they leave and return to the unit on the unit board.		
b. The staff will adhere to their assigned/designated break time.		
10. Assigns beds using telechecking responds in 15 minutes.		
11. Assigns meeting/inservice attendance and coverage as appropriate in collaboration with the Unit Manager or Administrative supervisor.		
12. Reports unusual occurrences, medication errors, on-the-job accidents, patient complaints and visitor illness, injury to Unit Manager/Assistant Unit Manager/Administrative Supervisor.		
13. Monitors the ADT log for accuracy of census in collaboration with the Unit Secretary and in their absence.		
14. Reviews sitter cases in collaboration with the Unit Manager/Patient Care Coordinator every shift. Documents sitter cases on assignment sheet.		
15. Clarifies policy and procedures and/or directs questions to the Unit Manager/Administrative Supervisor.		
16. Understand what is happening in whole hospital in order to adjust running the unit.		
17. Manage cost and supply issues.		

D. Human Relations Skills Competencies: *Responsibilities to interact effectively with other personnel to accomplish the requirements of patient care as well as administrative activities.* 1. Be accessible—identify self as the charge nurse.		
2. Influence atmosphere of unit in positive manner.		
3. Demonstrate caring for others.		
4. Communicate effectively with charge nurse, on-going/off-going shift, physicians, patient's families, staff, supervisors.		
5. Communicates with the on-coming/off-going charge nurse to convey patient care concerns/needs, staffing issues, and utilizes effective problem-solving skills in the delivery of nursing care.		
6. Communicates concerns to the Unit Manager/Administrative supervisor.		
7. Deals with difficult people, situations, shifts.		
8. Uses diplomacy with people.		
9. Gets along with people.		
10. Interacts positively with nurse manager.		
11. Provides leadership during the shift.		
12. Motivates staff to accomplish the mission.		
13. Protects staff.		
14. Addresses patient complaints, utilizing service recovery plan.		
15. Role-models effectively.		
16. Acts as a resource to the nursing staff (including agency nurses).		
17. Develop and train the staff.		
18. Supports staffs' personal needs.		
19. Team build—develop cooperative efforts.		
20. Assists in the development and maintenance of a supportive unit climate in which staff members respond to each other in a way that contributes to effective team building.		

ROLE—Role Related

Self-assessment	Evaluation/ validation methods	Levels	Type of validation	Comments
❏ Experienced ❏ Need practice ❏ Never done ❏ Not applicable (based on scope of practice)	❏ Verbal ❏ Demonstration/ observation ❏ Practical exercise ❏ Interactive class	❏ Beginner ❏ Intermediate ❏ Expert	❏ Orientation ❏ Annual ❏ Other _____	

Employee signature

Observer signature

ROLE—Role Related

Name: _____   Date: _____

Skill: **Defibrillator Function—Daily Check (Lifepak 9)**

Steps	Completed	Comments
1. Verifies paddles are firmly seated in test load (storage) area.		
2. Pushes 2 "energy select." Selects 200 joules if not already selected.		
3. Pushes 3 "charge." "Joules changing" will appear in lower right corner of monitor screen. Increasing numbers indicate energy level as defibrillator charges.		
4. Determines defibrillator is ready when the selected energy and the "joules available" messages appear in the lower right corner of monitor screen.		
5. Ascertains that "charge" button indicator light glows steadily and a charge complete tone is heard. Determines charge cycle takes ≤ 10 seconds.		
6. Pushes the apex discharge button only and verifies the unit does not discharge.		
7. Pushes the sternum discharge button only and verifies that unit does not discharge.		
8. Discharges defibrillator by pushing both paddle discharge buttons simultaneously.		
9. Verifies the message "test 200 joules delivered" appears in lower right corner of screen for three seconds.		
10. Retrieves recorder printout of "time, date, and defib test 200 joules delivered."		
11. Documents on daily log of defibrillator readiness for use.		

Self-assessment	Evaluation/ validation methods	Levels	Type of validation	Comments
❏ Experienced ❏ Need practice ❏ Never done ❏ Not applicable (based on scope of practice)	❏ Verbal ❏ Demonstration/ observation ❏ Practical exercise ❏ Interactive class	❏ Beginner ❏ Intermediate ❏ Expert	❏ Orientation ❏ Annual ❏ Other _____	

_____   _____
Employee signature   *Observer signature*

Evidence-Based Competency Management for the Medical-Surgical Unit, Second Edition

ROLE—Role Related

Name: _____ Date: _____

Skill: Discharge Bed/Bassinette Cleaning for Environmental Associates

Steps	Completed	Comments
1. Apply gloves. Use goggles if mixing concentrate.		
2. Mix germicidal cleaning solution, diluting concentrate correctly.		
3. Remove the pillow case from the pillow. Set aside. Remove the pillow case from the bassinette mattress.		
4. Carefully loosen the linen from the corners of the bed and roll toward the center of the bed to make a neat bundle. Place the rolled bundle of linen into the pillow case.		
5. Check the bedside table and the patient restroom for any wash cloths and bath towels so that they can be disposed of with the soiled linen.		
6. Wash bassinette.		
7. Wipe the patient's pillow with the cleaning cloth, which has been wrung out in the germicidal solution.		
8. Raise the head and foot of the bed by the remote switch.		
9. Wring out the cleaning cloth in the germicidal solution. Wipe down one half of the headboard, cleaning both front and back.		
10. Move on to wipe on half of the mattress and bed frame. Begin by wiping the top of the mattress.		
11. Wring out cleaning cloth in germicidal solution and wipe the bed frame and bedrails.		
12. For cleaning the footboard, follow the same cleaning procedure used on the headboard.		
13. After cleaning the other side of the mattress, headboard, bed frame, bedrails, and footboard, return the mattress to its normal position.		
14. Empty germicidal solution in restroom toilet.		
15. Get clean linen from linen closet.		
16. Make the bed.		

ROLE—Role Related

17. Set up room for next patient.				
Self-assessment	**Evaluation/ validation methods**	**Levels**	**Type of validation**	**Comments**
❏ Experienced ❏ Need practice ❏ Never done ❏ Not applicable (based on scope of practice)	❏ Verbal ❏ Demonstration/ observation ❏ Practical exercise ❏ Interactive class	❏ Beginner ❏ Intermediate ❏ Expert	❏ Orientation ❏ Annual ❏ Other _____	

_____   _____
Employee signature   *Observer signature*

Evidence-Based Competency Management for the Medical-Surgical Unit, Second Edition

ROLE—Role Related

Name: _____ Date: _____

Skill: HOP Charges

Steps	Completed	Comments
1. Identifies if patient is a 23 hour assign/HOP/EO or admitted.		
2. Identifies on the HOP patient (includes the patient's written assign or EO) the time the observation expires. At this time (or before this time), alerts the RN to notify the physician of the need for the admit order to be written.		
3. Identifies correct "Hourly Observation Charges form."		
4. Stamps form with the correct patient name plate.		
5. Records the date/time in (arrival time to the unit) and the date/time out (time patient was discharged from the unit, or transferred to ICU, SCVICU, or taken to the OR then admitted to another floor—use time the order was written; if no order written then use the time the patient left the observation floor).		
6. Calculates the difference from the time assigned to the time discharged/admitted. Rounds to the nearest hour (no minutes; i.e., if 1–29 minutes, drops the minute, keeps only the hour; if 30–59 minutes, then round to the next hour).		
7. Places the calculated hour amount in the correct unit line.		
8. Sends the form urgent mail to "data entry at Summa Center." Sends all forms from each unit together every morning.		
9. Delivers to the urgent mail box.		
10. Follows up with a status change form: if being discharged or being changed to an admitted patient, marks form accordingly and faxes to admitting.		

Self-assessment	Evaluation/ validation methods	Levels	Type of validation	Comments
❏ Experienced ❏ Need practice ❏ Never done ❏ Not applicable (based on scope of practice)	❏ Verbal ❏ Demonstration/ observation ❏ Practical exercise ❏ Interactive class	❏ Beginner ❏ Intermediate ❏ Expert	❏ Orientation ❏ Annual ❏ Other _____	

_____   _____
Employee signature   *Observer signature*

ROLE—Role Related

Name: _____ Date: _____

Skill: **Insurance Precertification Authorization**

Steps	Completed	Comments
1. Examines the chart for type of insurance.		
2. Determines if test needs precertified or authorized.		
3. Calls the phone number on the insurance card for benefits verification and authorization.		
4. Gives insurance company information regarding test ordered.		
5. Documents in chart: • Name of person spoke with at insurance company • Authorization number (if applicable)		
6. Enters authorization number into MPAC INVU screen.		
7. Identifies resource person if difficulties arise.		

Self-assessment	Evaluation/ validation methods	Levels	Type of validation	Comments
❏ Experienced ❏ Need practice ❏ Never done ❏ Not applicable (based on scope of practice)	❏ Verbal ❏ Demonstration/ observation ❏ Practical exercise ❏ Interactive class	❏ Beginner ❏ Intermediate ❏ Expert	❏ Orientation ❏ Annual ❏ Other _____	

_____   _____
Employee signature   *Observer signature*

Evidence-Based Competency Management for the Medical-Surgical Unit, Second Edition

ROLE—Role Related

Name: _____ Date: _____

Skill: **LPN Skills Assessment/Evaluation**

Steps	Completed	Comments
I. Competency A. Nursing Process 1. Assists RN in data collection, implementation, and evaluation of nursing care.		
2. Provides patient teaching.		
3. Prioritizes care for a group of patients.		
4. Utilizes appropriate resources.		
B. Technical Skills 1. Monitors/discontinues IVs.		
2. Maintains gastric/feeding tubes.		
3. Inserts/maintains urinary catheters.		
4. Performs trach care and suctioning.		
5. Assesses patient safety including proper utilization of restraints.		
6. Completes tissue therapy.		
7. Completes American Heart Association guidelines for BLS-Healthcare provider in CPR.		
8. Sets oxygen gauge rate.		
9. Locates various items on the emergency cart.		
10. Identifies nursing responsibilities in emergency situations.		
11. Provides and documents pre- and postop nursing care.		
12. Incorporates nursing measures to reduce and prevent the spread of infection in daily nursing care.		
13. Performs neurological checks when appropriate.		
14. Draws blood routine blood specimens.		
15. Performs BGT.		
16. Performs Blood Culture.		
17. Other		

C. Medications 1. Completes medication exam with a minimum score of 80%.		
2. Describes usual dose, common side effects, compatibilities, action, and untoward reactions of medications.		
3. Administers medications a. I.M.		
b. SQ and Insulin		
c. Calculations		
d. Other		
4. Documents administration of medication (MAR, controlled drugs, etc.)		
5. Identifies medication error reporting system.		
II. Accountability/Leadership A. Completes orientation statement of agreement.		
B. Accepts responsibilities as delegated.		
C. Follows appropriate employee policies and procedures, i.e. call off, time off, LOA, etc.		
D. Conforms to dress code.		
E. Identifies role of the nurse in quality assurance.		
F. Maintains safe working environment.		
G. Contains costs through proper use of supplies and maintenance of equipment.		
III. Communication A. Documents on the following forms: Interdisciplinary Assessment		
Graphic Record/PLATO.		
Interdisciplinary Progress Record		
Nursing Ongoing Assessment		
Unusual Occurrence		
B. Uses correct lines of communication.		
C. Attends Computer Class.		
D. Gives prompt, accurate, and pertinent report RN.		
E. Interacts with patients, significant others and health team members in positive manner.		

ROLE—Role Related

IV. Other A. Has completed Human Resources/Survey Orientation.		

Self-assessment	Evaluation/ validation methods	Levels	Type of validation	Comments
❏ Experienced ❏ Need practice ❏ Never done ❏ Not applicable (based on scope of practice)	❏ Verbal ❏ Demonstration/ observation ❏ Practical exercise ❏ Interactive class	❏ Beginner ❏ Intermediate ❏ Expert	❏ Orientation ❏ Annual ❏ Other _____	

_____   _____
Employee signature   *Observer signature*

ROLE—Role Related

Name: _____ Date: _____

Skill: Nursing Assistant Orientation Skills Assessment/Evaluation

Steps	Completed	Comments
A. Ability to do basic patient care as follows: Complete bed bath.		
Partial bath.		
Assists with shower.		
Oral hygiene (bid & prn).		
Back care.		
Peri care.		
Hair care.		
Offering/removal of bed pan or urinal.		
Ambulatory/assist to bathroom.		
Cath care.		
Documentation of output on bedside worksheet.		
Feeding patient, including compensatory strategies for feeding dysphagic patient.		
Assists patient with meeting all basic patient needs, toileting, walking, call light, etc.		
Makes Occupied bed.		
Makes Unoccupied bed.		
Accurately measures patient intake & output and records.		
Patient transfer/discharge.		
Supports safety of patient i.e. side rails, slippers or pt. lift, prn.		
Pneumatic Cuffs: Anti-embolic Therapy applied correctly.		
Uses hot (T-pad) and cold (ice) therapy safely.		
Uses **patient safety** properly, i.e., documentation of restraints.		
B. Communication skills Responds to call lights promptly.		
Anticipates & clarifies needs, i.e. pain, weakness, verbalizes to patient's nurse when needed.		

Evidence-Based Competency Management for the Medical-Surgical Unit, Second Edition

ROLE—Role Related

C. Provide age appropriate care 1. Recognizes need/independent decision-making (adults).		
2. Promotes bowel & bladder continence per toileting schedule.		
3. Provides privacy.		
4. Assist/orientation to room, equipment & surroundings.		
5. Removes dirty linen or equipment from patient room.		
D. Provides nutrition support 1. Passes and picks up trays, setting items up for ease of use.		
2. Records Intake (& output) accurately on worksheet in room.		
3. Identifies the percentage eaten of meals accurately in PLATO.		
4. Positions the patient for safety and comfort prior to eating.		
5. Encourages and assists with patient's meals, being aware of specific needs, and feeding patients as needed.		
E. Technical skills 1. BLS course: Heartsaver or Health Care Provider (optional).		
2. Assures patient's nurse is monitoring oxygen before & after activities (i.e. transport).		
3. Identifies responsibilities in emergency situations.		
4. Uses measures to reduce and prevent spread of infection in daily patient care.		
5. **Demonstrates ability to take and record vital signs** a. Takes **oral &/or axillary Temperature** & records.		
b. Use electronic automated blood pressure machine to take BP & records.		
c. Counts (30 seconds) & records **Radial pulse** rate accurately or records pulse from BP machine.		

d. Counts **respiratory rate** and records accurately.		
e. Reports variances, and patient needs to patient's Nurse for follow-up.		
F. Demonstrates ability to obtain and transport specimens 1. Sputum		
2. Urine/routine & CCMS		
3. Stool		
G. Body mechanics 1. Demonstrates proper lifting/turning/transferring patient techniques.		
2. Demonstrates proper technique in transferring patient from bed to cart and back.		
3. Uses proper positions & turning, protecting skin & bony prominences. Uses turning schedule.		
H. Environmental needs 1. Replaces trash bags, removes excess linen, etc. from rooms.		
2. Keeps pathways clear, free from clutter, checks lights, & other equipment in patient room.		
I. Performs postmortem care		
J. Assists with transport of patient to the morgue		
K. Safety 1. Verbalizes safety issues with equipment (step ladders, hand tools, light bulbs, etc.) to patient's nurse.		
2. Reports problems with lighting, equipment or supplies that cannot be repaired by nursing staff to maintenance.		
3. Identifies light maintenance duties.		
L. Demonstrates ability to **Contact Distribution** Department for needed patient care items.		
M. Unit Communication 1. Documents on patient chart on Nursing Treatment Record & PLATO accurately.		
2. Telephone/answers phone by identifying unit, name, & status.		

ROLE—Role Related

3. Operates pneumatic tube system/describes use (Class)		
4. Uses principles of patient confidentiality.		
5. Communicating to RN – any unusual observations (Signs and Symptoms) **PROMPTLY**.		
N. Interacts positively with patients, their significant others, and health team members.		
O. Punctuality 1. Arrives promptly in uniform.		
2. Notifies nursing office of absences by nursing policy.		
3. Notifies nursing office of lateness per policy.		
4. Notifies nurse in charge if leaving unit, returns promptly.		
P. Safety issues (Should be able to discuss and correctly answer questions on the following safety topics) 1. Fire Safety (Code Red)		
2. Bomb Threat (Code Black)		
3. Code Blue (Medical)		
4. Code Violet		
5. Infection Prevention & Exposure Control		
6. Disaster (Code Yellow)		
7. Evacuation		
8. Back Safety		
9. Severe Weather		
10. Electrical Safety		
11. Code Adam		
Q. Examinations 1. Standard precautions & Terminology		
2. Patient Safety		
3. Patient Limited Activity		
4. Hygiene		
R. SLPs		
S. Unit Competencies		

ROLE—Role Related

Self-assessment	Evaluation/ validation methods	Levels	Type of validation	Comments
❑ Experienced ❑ Need practice ❑ Never done ❑ Not applicable (based on scope of practice)	❑ Verbal ❑ Demonstration/ observation ❑ Practical exercise ❑ Interactive class	❑ Beginner ❑ Intermediate ❑ Expert	❑ Orientation ❑ Annual ❑ Other _____	

_____
Employee signature

_____
Observer signature

ROLE—Role Related

Name: _____ Date: _____

Skill: **Nursing Student Technician Competency Checklist**

Steps	Completed	Comments
A. Skills		
1. Basic care (bath, hair, teeth, ADLs).		
2. Ambulation.		
3. K-Pads.		
4. Ice bags.		
5. I & O documentation.		
6. Meal trays (administer & feed).		

7. Care of patient:
   a. With oxygen
   b. Stable postoperative
   c. With cast/splints (stable)		

8. Vital signs (BP, T, P, R).		

9. Obtain specimens
   a. Sputum
   b. Urine
   c. Stool		

10 Catheter care
   a. External male cath application
   b. Cath care		

11. Patient discharge (gather belongings & transfer).		

12. Team (CPR certification)
   a. Role in Team I
   b. dDefibrillation location (STH only)		

13. Morgue care (assist with care, transport body).		
14. Observational skills (reports s/s to RN).		
15. Transport patients, body mechanics, and transfer techniques.		
16. Transfer patients.		
17. Valuables procedure.		

18. Weights:
   a. Bedside
   b. Portable		

19. Documentation
    a. Graphics sheet
    b. Dietary intake
    c. I&O
    d. IPN		

20. Enema.		

21. Catheterization
    a. Straight
    b. Foley		

22. Sterile/nonsterile compress.		
23. Skin preps.		
24. Traction.		
25. Dressing changes.		
26. Trach care.		
27. Suctioning.		
28. Blood draws (Note: No blood draws from central lines or PICCs)		

Self-assessment	Evaluation/ validation methods	Levels	Type of validation	Comments
❏ Experienced ❏ Need practice ❏ Never done ❏ Not applicable (based on scope of practice)	❏ Verbal ❏ Demonstration/ observation ❏ Practical exercise ❏ Interactive class	❏ Beginner ❏ Intermediate ❏ Expert	❏ Orientation ❏ Annual ❏ Other _____	

_____   _____

Employee signature   *Observer signature*

ROLE—Role Related

Name: _____ Date: _____

Skill: **Private Duty RN/LPN Competency Evaluation**

Steps	Completed	Comments
1. Demonstrates professional appearance, behavior, and confidentiality.		
2. Follows established policies and procedures within Summa Health System.		
3. Maintains patient safety through knowledge of emergency codes and appropriate actions (i.e., evaluation maps/safe areas).		
4. Verbalize the location of emergency equipment and the knowledge of C.P.R. procedure.		
5. Communicates appropriately with patient, family, and staff.		
6. Reports to the Registered Nurse/Designee prior to leaving patient unattended and upon returning to the unit from breaks.		
7. Implements body Substance Isolation precautions.		
8. Documents accurate implementation and evaluation of patient care.		
9. Follows through with proper IV maintenance by documenting and reporting all elements of IV therapy. **(RN Only)**.		
10. Administers, documents, and evaluates all medications appropriately according to Summa Health System policies and procedures. **(RN Only)**.		

Self-assessment	Evaluation/validation methods	Levels	Type of validation	Comments
❏ Experienced ❏ Need practice ❏ Never done ❏ Not applicable (based on scope of practice)	❏ Verbal ❏ Demonstration/observation ❏ Practical exercise ❏ Interactive class	❏ Beginner ❏ Intermediate ❏ Expert	❏ Orientation ❏ Annual ❏ Other _____	

Employee signature   *Observer signature*

ROLE—Role Related

Name: _____ Date: _____

Skill: Registration

Steps	Completed	Comments
1. Greets patient/informs of need to gather information in manner consistent with house rules.		
2. Determines if patient has been previously registered within system; verifies birth date and Social Security number. If not previously registered, demonstrates knowledge registering new patient.		
3. Uses correct CPI number, continues through registration screens, asks pertinent questions, enters data.		
4. Demonstrates knowledge of using insurance master; identifies MC/MED/commercial insurance HMO/PPO.		
5. Demonstrates knowledge of Medicare secondary payer questionnaire asking patient-appropriate questions.		
6. Informs/requests patient to sign appropriate consent forms (i.e., surgical procedure, laser).		
7. Closes interview/registration with "thank you."		

Self-assessment	Evaluation/ validation methods	Levels	Type of validation	Comments
❏ Experienced ❏ Need practice ❏ Never done ❏ Not applicable (based on scope of practice)	❏ Verbal ❏ Demonstration/ observation ❏ Practical exercise ❏ Interactive class	❏ Beginner ❏ Intermediate ❏ Expert	❏ Orientation ❏ Annual ❏ Other _____	

_____   _____
Employee signature   *Observer signature*

Evidence-Based Competency Management for the Medical-Surgical Unit, Second Edition

ROLE—Role Related

Name: _____ Date: _____

Skill: RN Skills Assessment/Evaluation

Steps	Completed	Comments
I. Competency:		
A. Applies a systematic problem-solving approach in the implementation of nursing plans of care: 1. Uses nursing process to systematically assess, plan, implement, and evaluate nursing care.		
2. Provide/documents patient teaching/discharge planning.		
3. Involves patient/significant other in plan of care.		
4. Prioritizes nursing care for a group of patients.		
5. Initiates patient referrals as needed.		
6. Utilizes appropriate resources.		
B. Intravenous Therapy 1. Initiates intravenous.		
2. Monitors intravenous according to policy and procedure: a. Checks rate		
b. Assesses for signs and symptoms of complications		
c. Initiates PRN adapter		
3. Uses infusion pumps correctly: • PCA		
• Baxter		
4. Draws blood specimens: • Routine		
• Central line		
• Blood cultures		
5. Administers blood and blood components.		
6. Maintains central line/hyperalimentation.		
7. Applies/changes central line dressing.		
8. Administers IV medications (I.V.P.B. IV push).		
9. Documents administration of IV Therapy.		

10. Completes IV Therapy exam with a minimum score of 80%.		
C. Medication Administration 　1. Describes usual dose, common side effects, compatibilities, action, and untoward reactions of medications.		
2. Administers medications 　　a. I.M.		
b. SQ and Insulin.		
c. Calculations.		
d. Other.		
3. Documents administration of medications (MAR, controlled drugs, etc.).		
4. Identifies medication error reporting system.		
D. Treatment and Procedures 　1. Inserts and maintains gastric feeding tubes.		
2. Inserts and maintains urinary catheters.		
3. Performs trach care and suctioning.		
4. Assesses patient safety including proper utilization of restraints.		
5. Completes tissue therapy self-learning packet.		
6. Provides and documents pre- and postop nursing care.		
7. Incorporates nursing measures to reduce and prevent the spread of infection in daily nursing care.		
8. Completes American Heart Association guidelines for BLS-C in CPR.		
9. Changes oxygen gauge and sets rate.		
10. Locates various items on the emergency cart.		
11. Identifies nursing responsibilities in emergency situations.		
12. Completes: 　　a. Admission of a patient.		
b. Transfer of a patient.		
c. Discharge of a patient.		
13. Performs neurological checks when appropriate.		

ROLE—Role Related

14. Performs BGT.		
15. Other.		
II. Communication		
A. Documents on the following forms: Initial Interdisciplinary Assessment		
1. Graphic Record		
2. Interdisciplinary Progress Record		
3. Nursing Discharge/Patient Teaching		
4. Interdisciplinary Plan of Care		
5. Unusual Occurrence		
B. Transcribes physicians' orders.		
C. Takes verbal orders from physician.		
D. Uses correct lines of communication.		
E. Attends Computer Class.		
F. Gives prompt, accurate, and pertinent shift report.		
G. Interacts with patients significant others and health team members in positive manner.		
III. Accountability/Leadership		
A. Completes orientation statement of agreement.		
B. Delegates patient care to other personnel appropriately.		
C. Follows appropriate employee policies and procedures, i.e. call off, time off, LOA, etc.		
D. Conforms to dress code.		
E. Identifies role of the nurse in quality assurance.		
F. Maintains safe working environment.		
G. Contains costs through proper use of supplies and maintenance of equipment.		
IV. Other:		
A. Has completed Human Resource/Safety Orientation.		

ROLE—Role Related

Self-assessment	Evaluation/ validation methods	Levels	Type of validation	Comments
❏ Experienced ❏ Need practice ❏ Never done ❏ Not applicable (based on scope of practice)	❏ Verbal ❏ Demonstration/ observation ❏ Practical exercise ❏ Interactive class	❏ Beginner ❏ Intermediate ❏ Expert	❏ Orientation ❏ Annual ❏ Other _____	

_____   _____

Employee signature   *Observer signature*

ROLE—Role Related

Name: _____ Date: _____

Skill: **Sitter Guidelines/Expectations**

Steps	Completed	Comments
1. General Guidelines/Expectations Verbalizes or demonstrates: • Proper attire worn. • TV's and radios in patient's room are for the sole use of patient and not to be used by Float SA/Sitter Staff. • Food and beverages are not to be consumed in the patient's rooms.		
2. Lunches/Breaks/End of Shift Verbalizes or demonstrates: • Two (2) 15-minutes breaks and one half hour lunch during their 8-hour shift. • Break discussed with the RN responsible for the patient prior to starting their assignment. • Relief personnel present in the room before leaving for a break or lunch. • Use the call light to summon the nurse and ask for relief. If no relief at approved break and lunch. • **PATIENT NEVER LEFT ALONE UNTIL RELIEF PERSONNEL ARE AVAILABLE.** • Emergency requires sitter to leave the room at other than the scheduled break times, or if the next shift's sitter has not arrived by the end of your shift, summon the nurse, using the call light, to advise them that you need to leave the room. • Returning from lunch or break, reports to the Nursing Station to let them know of return.		

3. Patient Care Guidelines Verbalizes or demonstrates: • **DO NOT LEAVE THE PATIENT ATTENDED.** • Family visiting and asks sitter to leave the room. Stay in the immediate area of the patient's room so that you are aware of when the family leaves. A chair can be placed in the hall by the door to sit in while the family is visiting. • **DOES NOT SLEEP WHILE ON DUTY.** • Remain by the patient's bedside to assist them when taking fluids and nourishment, if permitted or directed, and to protect the patient from injury. • Does not comment or discuss patient or the family/visitors issues related to the patient's care, conditions or concerns about the nursing staff. • Alter to any change in the patient's behavior or condition (such as their breathing pattern, vomiting, restlessness, perspiring, pain or other signs or symptoms of difficulty and report these to unit personnel immediately. **Uses the call light to summon unit personnel immediately.**			
4. Patient Care Responsibilities Verbalized or demonstrates: • Assists the unit staff to change the bed linens and patient's gown if necessary. • Provides assistant to the unit staff with patient's shower or bath. • Assists patient with personal hygiene such as brushing their teeth, washing face and hands, etc. • Assists unit staff to turn patient when requested. • Under the direction of the nursing staff, assists the patient into a chair or to the bathroom. Float SA/Sitter is to remain with patient and assist them back to bed. • Intervenes to prevent patient from falling and pulling at tubes. If a patient falls, if it becomes difficult to keep patient from pulling their IV or tubes, or if it appears that a tube has been pulled out of place **UNIT STAFF SUMMONED IMMEDIATELY.** • Assists the patient with the bedpan or urinal as necessary. Measure urine output and report to the Nurse if so directed.			

Evidence-Based Competency Management for the Medical-Surgical Unit, Second Edition

ROLE—Role Related

5. Patient with Suicide Precautions
   Verbalized or demonstrates:
   - Restricts patient to his/her own room. Patient should not leave the room without constant staff accompaniment (i.e., diagnostic tests, treatments). **Accompany the patient off the unit. At no time is the patient to be out of your or another staff member's vision.**
   - Patient wears a hospital gown at all times.
   - Removes potentially hazardous items from the patient's environment. This includes, but is not limited to: alcoholic beverages, cleaning solutions, crochet hooks, electrical appliances, glass items, glass vases, hangers, knitting needles, knives, lighters, lotions, matches, medications, metal eating utensils, nail polish remover, needles/sharps containers, perfume, picture frames, pins, plastic bags, pop cans, razor blades, scissors, spray containers, thumb tacks, tweezers.
   - Surveys the environment for any restricted items.
   - **Restricted items may be used ONLY in the presence of a staff member.**
   - Reminds visitors not to leave potentially harmful items with the patient.
   - **Patients are not to be out of the sitter's vision when visitors are present.**
   - Patient belongings placed in a bag, labeled, and either sent home with the family or kept at nurse's station until patient's discharge.
   - Meal Tray Precautions:
     a. **Paper tray set-up** through dietary.
     b. When serves a patient, assure that paper cups and plates and plastic utensils are on the tray both before and after meals. Cuts food and remove the knife and fork. Finger foods OK.
     c. Reports any missing items to the Registered Nurse.
   - Patients are not permitted to wander in the hall. Report patient leaving room to RN. Don't lose sight of the patient.
   - Patients are not permitted to leave the unit AMA.

ROLE—Role Related

Self-assessment	Evaluation/ validation methods	Levels	Type of validation	Comments
❑ Experienced ❑ Need practice ❑ Never done ❑ Not applicable (based on scope of practice)	❑ Verbal ❑ Demonstration/ observation ❑ Practical exercise ❑ Interactive class	❑ Beginner ❑ Intermediate ❑ Expert	❑ Orientation ❑ Annual ❑ Other _____	

_____   _____
Employee signature   *Observer signature*

ROLE—Role Related

Name: _____   Date: _____

Skill: **Telephone Skills**

Steps	Completed	Comments
1. Answers the telephone in three rings or less.		
2. Identifies self by department, title, and name in appropriate professional business tone and language.		
3. Asks caller how one can be of service (example: "How may I help you today?").		
4. Demonstrates placing caller on hold, checking back every 30 seconds or less while looking for additional information for the caller.		
5. Demonstrates transferring a call when the caller has accessed one's department incorrectly.		
6. Demonstrates taking a message: records caller's name, nature of message, telephone number, etc.		
7. Closes conversation with offers of any other assistance and thank you.		

Self-assessment	Evaluation/ validation methods	Levels	Type of validation	Comments
❏ Experienced ❏ Need practice ❏ Never done ❏ Not applicable (based on scope of practice)	❏ Verbal ❏ Demonstration/ observation ❏ Practical exercise ❏ Interactive class	❏ Beginner ❏ Intermediate ❏ Expert	❏ Orientation ❏ Annual ❏ Other _____	

_____   _____

Employee signature   *Observer signature*

Name: _____ Date: _____

Skill: Telephone Skills (Problem Solving)

Steps	Completed	Comments
1. Answers routine telephone calls by the third ring in a friendly manner by identifying his or her name and department.		
2. Refers to interdepartmental phone book and class schedules to help locate any employees or meetings in our buildings. Asks for clarification.		
3. Utilizes other staff members for telephone coverage while away from the desk area/has someone sit at the reception desk to cover the phone calls.		
4. Before leaving for lunch or break, asks who is available to cover the phone. Gives a time reference as to when he or she is leaving and will be returning.		
5. Notifies person when he or she returns.		
6. Keeps Rolodex up-to-date.		
7. Retrieves voicemail message in a timely manner and responds/follows through accordingly.		

Self-assessment	Evaluation/ validation methods	Levels	Type of validation	Comments
❏ Experienced ❏ Need practice ❏ Never done ❏ Not applicable (based on scope of practice)	❏ Verbal ❏ Demonstration/ observation ❏ Practical exercise ❏ Interactive class	❏ Beginner ❏ Intermediate ❏ Expert	❏ Orientation ❏ Annual ❏ Other _____	

_____ _____
Employee signature *Observer signature*

ROLE—Role Related

Name: _____ Date: _____

Skill: **Unit Secretary Orientation Skills Assessment/Evaluation**

Steps	Completed	Comments
I. Clinical Duties A. Transcription 1. Correctly identifies and transcribes/processes stat or other priority orders into PLATO.		
2. Correctly transcribes current medication orders onto the Medication Administration Record (MAR): • Processes orders from paper to PLATO. • Sends Home Medication List & Order sheet to Pharmacy if needed.		
3. Correctly transcribes Lab orders by: a. Completing requisitions, if needed. b. Notifying Nursing, and printing lab labels, placing in biohazard bag. c. Processing in PLATO, creating ADT logs, or other lists as unit appropriate.		
4. Correctly transcribes other Diagnostic orders and other physician consultations. a. (Radiology, Cardiology, Neurology Testing, etc.) • Completing Diagnostic Requisitions. b. Scheduling the diagnostic studies. 1) Calling physician office and/or 2) Clinical diagnostic test unit. c. Adding consulting physician to the patient provider list PLATO. d. Sending Notification of Added Physician message in (PLATO). e. Printing the appropriate Prep slips.		
5. Correctly transcribes Respiratory orders by accurately: a. Notifying Respiratory Therapy. b. Recording order on PLATO.		
6. Correctly transcribes Dietary orders by: a. Recording the order on the Diet Roster.		

b. Notifying Dietary of late orders.		
7. Correctly transcribes treatment orders by accurately: a. Entering order to PLATO.		
b. Notifying the department or technician of the order per flow-sheet procedure, if not automatically done in PLATO (i.e., Nutrition Support, RT or EKG).		
c. Ordering the appropriate patient care equipment.		
B. Manages patient chart assembly as required. 1. Admission		
2. Discharge		
3. Transfer • Sends PLATO message (Registration). • Notifies RN to create a current list of orders to be used on receiving unit (non-PLATO to PLATO).		
4. Pre/PostOp • Checklist review. • Generates patient information sheets, if available.		
5. Thinning charts (to "older" sections on unit). • Correctly removes only what is allowed to be thinned. • Recollates charts into one medical record at discharge.		
C. Notifies Patient Registration of Admissions, discharges, deaths, transfers or change of status. • Using Status Change Form. • Using PLATO system, when available.		
D. Completes chart rounds including: 1. Checks charts adding additional forms.		
2. Assures correct chart order.		
3. Places MAR's, reports or transfer record, etc., on chart in correct location.		
E. Sorts incoming mail/faxes and files in appropriate charts.		
F. Uses and files OR, Radiology, PT or other schedules as appropriate resources.		

ROLE—Role Related

G. Completes and updates, as appropriate: 1. Supervisor's Report or Optilink™ review.		
2. Dietary Roster, sending messages to Dietary or phoning with updated information.		
3. Daily Work List (i.e., form 90200150) if used.		
4. ADT Log.		
5. Consult Log.		
6. Communication Board.		
7. Bulletin Boards.		
8. Routine Labs (serial and daily).		
9. Census Check in OptiLink™.		
10. Central Transport list of transfers.		
11. Shift Flags turned on and off in PLATO.		
12. **Other unit-based competencies as required.**		
H. Demonstrate Use of 1. Telephone (Desk and Electronic)		
2. Patient Intercom		
3. Page System		
4. Pneumatic Tube		
5. Lab Label Printer & Addressograph imprinter		
6. Copy Machine		
7. Care Windows Class/PLATO Class		
8. Central Transport In-Patient Request call Notification of Transfer (to unit or morgue) • Enters Medical Record # without extra 00s		
9. E-mail class		
10. Fax Machine		
• Adding paper		
• Adding toner		
II. Clerical Duties A. Orders office supplies as needed.		
B. Orders forms as needed.		
III. Examination Completes the Medical Terminology exam with a minimum score of 80%.		
IV. Basic Lift Support (Circle One) **HeartSaver CPR Health Care Provider**		

V. Communication		
1. Reads email and prints communication to staff / places on unit bulletin board as needed.		
2. Sends pager text message and receives feedback from person paged.		
3. Documents a page returned on Consult Lob.		
VI. Human Relations A. Gives prompt, accurate, shift report to on-coming unit secretary		
B. Arrives on time in uniform.		
C. Notifies Nursing Administration Office and unit of absenteeism according to policy.		
D. Notifies unit manager and nursing administration office of tardiness according to policy.		
E. Notifies nurse in charge when leaving unit consistently.		
F. Follows current guidelines for breaks and lunch.		
G. Emails Staff Development Instructor with preceptor's name.		
VIII. Personal Appearance A. Conforms to dress code.		
IX. Completes self-learning packets as appropriate:		
New Employee Orientation		
MOE: • Fire/Electrical Safety • Evacuation • Hazard Communication • Infection Control • Weather Emergencies • Codes: Adam, Black, Blue, Red, Violet, Yellow		
X. Knows Armband colors • High Risk Falls armband alert • Allergy • Admission		

ROLE—Role Related

Self-assessment	Evaluation/ validation methods	Levels	Type of validation	Comments
❏ Experienced ❏ Need practice ❏ Never done ❏ Not applicable (based on scope of practice)	❏ Verbal ❏ Demonstration/ observation ❏ Practical exercise ❏ Interactive class	❏ Beginner ❏ Intermediate ❏ Expert	❏ Orientation ❏ Annual ❏ Other _____	

_____   _____
Employee signature   *Observer signature*

Bibliography

General

Alvare, S., Dugan, D., and Fuzy, J. 2005. *Nursing Assistant Care.* Albuquerque, NM: Hartman Publishing.

American College of Cardiology and the American Heart Association 2004. *ACC/AHA Guideline for the Management of Patients With ST-Elevation Myocardial Infarction Pocket Guide.*

American Geriatrics Society, British Geriatrics Society, and American Academy of Orthopaedic Surgeons Panel on Falls Prevention. 2001. Guidelines for the prevention of falls in older persons. *Journal of the American Geriatrics Society* 49(5): 664-672.

American Heart Association. 2005. American Heart Association guidelines for cardiopulmonary resuscitation and emergency cardiovascular care. *Circulation* 112: IV35-IV46.

Brunt, B. 2007. *Competencies for Staff Educators: Tools to Evaluate and Enhance Nursing Professional Development.* Marblehead, MA: HCPro, Inc.

Doloresco, L., Lloyd, T., Smith, L., and Weinel, D. 2002. A clinical evaluation of ceiling lifts: Lifting and transfer technology for the future. *SCI Nurse* 19(2): 75-77.

Duell, D., Martin, B., and Smith, S. 2008. *Clinical Nursing Skills: Basic to Advanced Skills.* 7th ed. Upper Saddle River, NJ: Pearson Education, Inc.

Gazmuri, R. et al. 2007. Scientific knowledge gaps and clinical research priorities for cardiopulmonary resuscitation and emergency cardiac care identified during the 2005 international consensus conference on E and CPR science with treatment recommendations: A consensus statement from the International Liaison Committee on Resuscitation, the American Heart Association Emergency Cardiovascular Care Committee, the Stroke Council and Cardiovascular Nursing Council. *Circulation* 116: 2501-2512.

National Heart Lung and Blood Institute. 2007. *Deep Vein Thrombosis.* United States Department of Health and Human Services.

Bibliography

Nissen, S., Pepine, C., Bashore, T., et al. 1994. American College of Cardiology position statement. Cardiac angiography without cine film: erecting a "tower of Babel" in the cardiac catheterization laboratory. *Journal of the American College of Cardiology* 24: 834-837.

Perry, A. and Potter, P. 2006. *Clinical Nursing Skills & Techniques.* 6th Ed. St. Louis, MO: Mosby.

Studer, Q. 2003. *Hardwiring Excellence.* Gulf Breeze, FL: Fire Starter Publishing.

United States Department of Labor Occupational Safety and Health Administration. Fit testing guidelines. Standards 29CFR 1910.134, Appendix A.

Urdern, L., Stacy, K., and Lough, M., eds. 2006. *Thelan's Critical Care Nursing: Diagnosis and Management.* 5th ed. St. Louis, MO: Mosby Elsevier.

Weinstein, S. 2007. *Plumer's Principles and Practice of Intravenous Therapy.* 8th ed. Philadelphia, PA: Lippincott.

Medical-Surgical

AABB. 2006. *Standards for Blood Bank and Transfusions.* 24th ed. Bethesda, MD: AABB.

Alvare, S., Dugan, D., and Fuzy, J. 2005. *Nursing Assistant Care.* Albuquerque, NM: Hartman Publishing.

American Diabetes Association. 2003. Position statement on insulin administration. *Diabetes Care* 26 (Supp. 1): 121.

American Heart Association. 2005. *BLS for Healthcare Providers.* Dallas, TX: AHA.

American Ophthalmological Society. 2003. *AOS Task Force on Curriculum in Ophthalmology for Medical Students.*

American Physical Therapy Association. 2007. *Standards of Practice for Physical Therapy.* Alexandria, VA: American Physical Therapy Association.

American Society for Gastrointestinal Endoscopy. 2002. Complications of upper GI endoscopy. *Gastrointestinal Endoscopy* 55(7): 784-793.

Bibliography

Asakura, T., et al. 2006. Handling and safety of two insulin injection pens (FlexPen® and OptiClik®) in insulin-naïve type 2 diabetic patients. *Diabetes* 55 (Supp. 1): A457.

Atrium Medical Corporation. 1993. *Managing Chest Drainage.* Hudson, NH: Atrium Medical Corporation.

Barthel, D., and Mahoney, F. 1965. Functional evaluation: the Barthel Index. *Maryland State Medical Journal* 14: 56-61.

Batirel, H., Lacin, T., Yildizeli, F., and Yuksel, M. 2004. Complications and management of long-term central venous access catheters and ports. *Journal of Vascular Access* 5(4): 174-178.

Berstrom, et al. 1994. *Treatment of Pressure Ulcers.* U.S. Department of Health and Human Service.

Black, et al. 2007. National Pressure Ulcer Advisory Panel's Updated Ulcer Staging System. *Urology Nursing* 27(2): 144-150.

Brennan, F., et al. 2007. The athletic preparticipation evaluation: cardiovascular assessment. *American Family Physician* 75: 1008-1014.

Bryan, R. 1997. Administering conscious sedation: Operational guidelines. *Critical Care Nursing Clinics of North America* 9(3): 289-300.

Byun, S., et al. 2003. Three dimension ultrasound bladder scanner predicts bladder volumes with good accuracy. *Urology* 62: 656-660.

Carlson, K. and Weigand, D. 2005. *AACN Procedure Manual for Critical Care.* 5th ed. St. Louis, MO: Elsevier Saunders.

Castaldi, P. 2005. *Clinical nursing skills and techniques.* 6th ed. St. Louis, MO: Elsevier Mosby.

Centers for Disease Control and Prevention. 2003. *Mantoux Tuberculin Skin Testing Training Materials Kit.*

Colyar, M. and Ehrhardt, C. 2001. *Ambulatory Care Procedures for the Nurse Practitioner.* Philadelphia, PA: F. A. Davis Company. 94-104.

Bibliography

Cooley, C. and Morgan, G. 2005. Injection system for two luteinizing hormone-releasing hormone agonists: A comparative assessment of administration times and nurses' perceptions. *European Journal of Oncology Nursing* 9(4): 334-340.

Diagnostic Ultrasound. 2001. *Urology for Primary Care.*

Duell, D., Martin, B., and Smith, S. 2008. *Clinical Nursing Skills: Basic to Advanced Skills. 7th ed.* Upper Saddle River, NJ: Pearson Education, Inc.

Fertig, B., Martin, D., and Simmons, D. 1995. Therapy for diabetes. *Diabetes in America.* 2nd ed. Bethesda, MD: National Institutes of Health. 519-540.

Infusion Nurses Society. 2006. *Infusion Nursing Standards of Practice.* Norwood, MA: Infusion Nurses Society.

The Joint Commission. 2006. *Tubing Misconnections – a persistent and potentially deadly occurrence.* www.jointcommission.org (retrieved May 25, 2006).

Joint Commission Resources. 2007. *Comprehensive Accreditation Manual for Hospitals: The Official Handbook.* Chicago, IL: The Joint Commission.

Kala, T., Matsuno, Y., Sekino, S., Takagi, H., and Umemoto, T. 2007. Intraoperative autotransfusion in abdominal aortic aneurysm surgery: Meta-analysis of randomized controlled trials. *Archives of Surgery* 142(11): 1098-1101.

McCall, R. and Tankersley, C. 2007. *Phlebotomy Essentials.* 4th ed. Philadelphia, PA: Lippincott Williams & Wilkins.

National Association of Orthopaedic Nurses. *Guidelines for Orthopaedic Nursing.* www.orthonurse.org (accessed January 28, 2008).

National Institute of Health. National Institute of Neurological Disorders and Stroke. http://www.ninds.nih.gov/index.htm (accessed February 12, 2008).

National Kidney Foundation. Clinical Practice Guidelines. www.kidney.org/professionals/doqi/guidelines/doqiupvai.html#doqiupva3 (accessed January 2007).

Norfolk Medical Products, Inc. 2003. *Aqua-C Hydration System Resource Guide.* Skokie, IL: Norfolk Medical Products, Inc.

Oncology Nursing Society (ONS). 2004. *Access Device Guidelines: recommendations for nursing practice and education.* 2nd ed. Pittsburgh, PA: Oncology Nursing Society.

Oncology Nursing Society. 2005. *Chemotherapy and Biotherapy Guidelines and Recommendations for Practice.* 2nd ed. Pittsburgh, PA: Oncology Nursing Society.

Perry, A. and Potter, P. 2006. *Clinical Nursing Skills & Techniques.* 6th Ed. St. Louis, MO: Mosby Elsevier.

Perry, A. and Potter, P. 2006. *Fundamentals of Nursing.* 6th ed. St. Louis, MO: Mosby Elsevier.
Roman, M. 2005. Tracheostomy tubes. *MedSurg Nursing* 14(2): 143-145.

Sasson, M. and Shvartzman, P. 2001. Hypodermoclysis: An alternative infusion technique. *American Family Physician* 64(9): 1575-1578.

Scibal, J. 2005. Control your schedule. Optometric management: June 2005.

September-October 2001. Patient-controlled analgesic infusion pumps: Evaluating the Deltec CADD-Prizm PCS II. *Health Devices* 30(9-10): 360-364.

Springhouse Corporation. 2004. *Nursing Procedures.* 4th ed. Philadelphia, PA: Lippincott Williams & Wilkin.

Summa Health System. *Patient Care Services Policy and Procedure Manual: Insulin Self-Administration.*

United States Department of Transportation. *Best Practices for DOT Random Drug and Alcohol Testing.* Office of the Secretary and Office of Drug and Alcohol Policy and Compliance.

Weinstein, S. 2007. *Plumer's Principles and Practice of Intravenous Therapy.* 8th ed. Philadelphia, PA: Lippincott.

Wiseman, J. 1998. *Standard Procedures for the Collection of Diagnostic Blood Specimens by Venipuncture.* 4th ed. Wayne, PA: National Committee for Clinical Laboratory Standards.

Nursing education instructional guide

Target audience:

- Chief nursing officer
- Chief nurse executive
- Directors of nursing
- Directors of nursing education
- VPs of nursing
- Nurse managers
- Staff educators
- Staff development specialist
- Human resource professional

Statement of need:

Organizations have to conduct regular staff competency assessments, and fulfilling Joint Commission competency requirements are a key part of the staff education role. As evidence-based practice has become the norm for nursing, educators are looking for competency assessments that are based on evidence. The second edition of this book ensures competencies are based on best evidence.

Educational objectives:

Upon completion of this activity, participants should be able to:

- Design a competency plan to effectively assess employee competence
- Identify advantages of competency-based education
- Describe methods of validating competencies
- Recognize the benefits of incorporating competency assessment into job descriptions and performance evaluation tools

Nursing education instructional guide

- Discuss the key elements required of performance-based job descriptions
- Develop a training program to train staff to perform competency assessment
- Maintain consistency in a competency validation system
- Identify steps for effective program documentation
- Recognize the essential qualities needed by competency assessors
- List potential categories for new competencies
- Identify best practices for implementing new competencies
- Discuss dimensions of competencies
- Differentiate between orientation checklists and skill checklists

Faculty:
Barbara A. Brunt, MA, MN, RN-BC
Adrianne E. Avillion, DEd, RN
Gwen A. Valois, MS, RN, BC
Jane G. Alberico, MS, RN, CEN

Accreditation/designation statement:
This educational activity for three contact hours is provided by HCPro, Inc. HCPro, Inc. is accredited as a provider of continuing nursing education by the American Nurses Credentialing Center's Commission on Accreditation.

Disclosure statements:
Barbara A. Brunt, Adrianne E. Avillion, Gwen A. Valois, and Jane G. Alberico have declared that they have no commercial/financial vested interest in this activity.

Instructions:
In order to be eligible to receive your nursing contact hour(s) for this activity, you are required to do the following:

Nursing education instructional guide

1. Read the book
2. Complete the exam
3. Complete the evaluation
4. Provide your contact information in the space provided on the exam and evaluation
5. Submit the exam and evaluation to HCPro, Inc.

Please provide all of the information requested above and mail or fax your completed exam, program evaluation, and contact information to:

> HCPro, Inc.
> ATTN: Continuing Education Department
> 200 Hoods Lane
> Marblehead, MA 01945
> Tel: 877/727-1728
> Fax: 781/639-2982

Nursing education exam

Name: _____

Title: _____

Facility name: _____

Address: _____

Address: _____

City: _____ State: _____ ZIP: _____

Phone number: _____ Fax number: _____

E-mail: _____

Nursing license number: _____

(ANCC requires a unique identifier for each learner)

1. When designing a competency plan, attention must be paid to all of the following except:

    a. The needs of the patients and families

    b. The extended community

    c. Former standards of practice

    d. Organizational policies and procedures

2. "Competent" can be defined as:

    a. Well-qualified, capable, fit

    b. Underqualified, weak

    c. Underachieving

    d. Levelheaded

3. Which of the following is not a benefit of a competency-based approach?

    a. Reducing staff anxiety

    b. Increasing staff retention

    c. Encouraging independence instead of teamwork

    d. Enhancing skills and knowledge

4. Competency involves what domains of practice?

   a. Cognitive, affective, and psychomotor

   b. Cognitive, disaffective, and psychomotor

   c. Cognitive, affective, and psychosomatic

   d. Intuitive, affective, and psychosomatic

5. All of the following are methods for validating competency except:

   a. Posttests

   b. Case studies

   c. Simulated events

   d. Estimations

6. Observations of daily work to ensure competency can include:

   a. Patient rounds

   b. Phone calls

   c. Staff conversations

   d. Family discussions

7. Which of the following is not a benefit of incorporating competency assessment into job descriptions and performance evaluation tools?

   a. Improved efficiency

   b. Improved patient safety

   c. Improved employee satisfaction

   d. Improved nurse/physician communication

Nursing education instructional guide

8. Practice standards in a well-developed competency- or performance-based job description should be:

   a. Subjective

   b. Measurable and objective

   c. Vague to interpretation

   d. Age-specific

9. When incorporating competency-based performance standards in job descriptions, sections should be devoted to all of the following except:

   a. Teamwork

   b. Mandatory safety requirements

   c. Communication

   d. Independence

10. Which of the following is not a component of a competency assessment training and education program?

    a. Purpose

    b. Learning styles

    c. Maintaining objectivity

    d. Withholding criticism

11. All of the following are principles of adult learning except:

    a. Adults must have a valid reason for learning

    b. Adults do not bring life experiences to a learning situation

    c. Adults are self-directed learners

    d. Adults respond to both extrinsic and intrinsic motivators

12. Consistency in documentation:

   a. is as important as consistency in approach

   b. is not as important as consistency in approach

   c. does not relate to consistency in approach

   d. results in consistency in approach

13. All of the following are common job titles that may carry with them the responsibility for competency assessment except:

   a. Preceptor

   b. Nurse manager

   c. Staff development specialist

   d. Unit secretary

14. To keep your validation system consistent, you should always maintain _____.

   a. Subjectivity

   b. Objectivity

   c. Biases

   d. Partiality

15. Which of the following is not a qualification a competency assessor should possess?

   a. Mediocre performance of the competencies being evaluated

   b. The desire to acquire or enhance adult education skills

   c. Demonstration of excellent interpersonal communication skills

   d. Tact and the desire to help colleagues improve their job performance

Nursing education instructional guide

16. What is not an essential component of competency documentation?

    a. Assessment documentation must be dated.

    b. Identify the specific competency being assessed.

    c. Identify the objectives that must be achieved to demonstrate competency.

    d. Document nonspecific steps in competency achievement.

17. All of the following are potential categories for new competencies except:

    a. New medications

    b. Old equipment

    c. Interpersonal communications

    d. New patient populations

18. What is not a best practice for implementing new competencies?

    a. Competency skills fairs

    b. Drills

    c. Self-assessment

    d. Word of mouth

19. The three dimensions of competencies include:

    a. Critical-thinking dimension, interpersonal dimension, and technical dimension

    b. Critical-thinking dimension, selective dimension, and scientific dimension

    c. Cognitive-thinking dimension, selective dimension, and technical dimension

    d. Correlated dimension, interpersonal dimension, and scientific dimension

20. The purpose of a competency program is to do all of the following except:

   a. Improve job performance

   b. Decrease organizational effectiveness

   c. Enhance patient outcomes

   d. Promote economic efficiency

21. Orientation checklists specify the ___, ____, and ____ needed to perform safely.

   a. techniques, abilities, and background

   b. intelligence, opinions, and viewpoints

   c. methods, talents, and capabilities

   d. knowledge, attitudes, and skills

22. Skills checklists should be:

   a. Learner oriented

   b. Unfocused on behaviors

   c. Ambiguous

   d. Immeasurable

Nursing education evaluation

Name: _____

Title: _____

Facility name: _____

Address: _____

Address: _____

City: _____ State: _____ ZIP: _____

Phone number: _____ Fax number: _____

E-mail: _____

Nursing license number: _____

(ANCC requires a unique identifier for each learner)

1. This activity met the following learning objectives:

a.) Designed a competency plan to effectively assess employee competence

    Strongly disagree   1   2   3   4   5   Strongly agree

b.) Identified advantages of competency-based education

    Strongly disagree   1   2   3   4   5   Strongly agree

c.) Determined methods of validating competencies

    Strongly disagree   1   2   3   4   5   Strongly agree

d.) Recognized the benefits of incorporating competency assessment into job descriptions and performance evaluation tools

    Strongly disagree   1   2   3   4   5   Strongly agree

e.) Discussed the key elements required of performance-based job descriptions

    Strongly disagree   1   2   3   4   5   Strongly agree f.) Developed a training program to train staff to perform competency assessment

    Strongly disagree   1   2   3   4   5   Strongly agree

g.) Maintained consistency in a competency validation system

    Strongly disagree   1   2   3   4   5   Strongly agree

h.) Identified steps for effective program documentation

    Strongly disagree   1   2   3   4   5   Strongly agree

i.) Recognized the essential qualities needed by competency assessors

    Strongly disagree   1   2   3   4   5   Strongly agree

j.) Listed potential categories for new competencies

    Strongly disagree   1   2   3   4   5   Strongly agree

k.) Identified best practices for implementing new competencies

    Strongly disagree   1   2   3   4   5   Strongly agree

l.) Discussed dimensions of competencies

    Strongly disagree   1   2   3   4   5   Strongly agree

m.) Differentiated between orientation checklists and skill checklists

    Strongly disagree   1   2   3   4   5   Strongly agree

2. *Objectives were related to the overall purpose/goal of the activity.*

    Strongly disagree   1   2   3   4   5   Strongly agree

Nursing education instructional guide

3. This activity was related to my nursing activity needs.

    Strongly disagree   1   2   3   4   5   Strongly agree

4. The exam for the activity was an accurate test of the knowledge gained.

    Strongly disagree   1   2   3   4   5   Strongly agree

5. The activity avoided commercial bias or influence.

    Strongly disagree   1   2   3   4   5   Strongly agree

6. This activity met my expectations.

    Strongly disagree   1   2   3   4   5   Strongly agree

7. Will this learning activity enhance your professional nursing practice?

    Yes   No

8. This educational method was an appropriate delivery tool for the nursing/clinical audience.

    Strongly disagree   1   2   3   4   5   Strongly agree

9. How committed are you to making the behavioral changes suggested in this activity?

    a. Very committed

    b. Somewhat committed

    c. Not committed

10. Please provide us with your degree.

    a. ADN

    b. BSN

    c. MSN

    d. Other, please state

11. Please provide us with your credentials.

   a. LVN

   b. LPN

   c. RN

   d. NP

   e. Other, please state

12. Providing nursing contact hours for this product influenced my decision to buy it.

   Strongly disagree   1   2   3   4   5   Strongly agree

13. I found the process to obtain my continuing education credits for this activity easy to complete.

   Strongly disagree   1   2   3   4   5   Strongly agree

14. If you did not find the process easy to complete, which of the following areas did you find the most difficult?

   a. Understanding the content of the activity

   b. Understanding the instructions

   c. Completing the exam

   d. Completing the evaluation

   e. Other, please state:

15. How much time did it take for you to complete this activity (this includes reading the book and completing the exam and the evaluation)? _____
_____

Nursing education instructional guide

16. If you have any comments on this activity, process, or selection of topics for nursing CE, please note them below.

_____

_____

_____

_____

17. Would you be interested in participating as a pilot tester for the development of future HCPro nursing education activities?

     Yes   No

Thank you for completing this evaluation of our nursing CE activity!